Bump It Up

Transform Your Pregnancy into the Ultimate Style Statement

Amy Tara Koch

BALLANTINE BOOKS

NEW YORK

A Ballantine Books Trade Paperback Original

Copyright © 2010 by Amy Tara Koch
Interior illustrations not otherwise credited are copyright © 2010
by Annika Wester/CWC International, Inc.

Published in the United States by Ballantine Books, an imprint of
The Random House Publishing Group, a division of Random House, Inc., New York.

BALLANTINE and colophon are registered trademarks of Random House, Inc.

ISBN 978-0-345-51447-9

Printed in the United States of America on acid-free paper

www.ballantinebooks.com

9 8 7 6 5 4 3 2 1

Book design by Vivian Ghazarian, Modern Good

Dedicated to the babes
who supplied me with
the most bewitching of bumps,
Isabella and Brette

CONTENTS

Introduction: From Miu Miu to Muumuu   ix

Preggo Glossary   xix

FIRST TRIMESTER:
Bloated on the Bias   1

SECOND TRIMESTER:
Channel Your Inner Fashion Editor   45

THIRD TRIMESTER:
Large and In Charge   137

FOURTH TRIMESTER:
Lighten Up!   161

Keeping It All Together   183

Acknowledgments   184

Resources   185

From Miu Miu to Muumuu

In the beginning there were
skinny jeans. Body-skimming knits
cavorted with tailored
trousers and thigh-grazing
dresses in the streams and valleys.
Silky G-strings and
non-industrial-sized support bras
tilled the fields. Stilettos roamed
the earth. And it was good.
Then came pregnancy.
Slim-cut ensembles were cast
from Eden. Muumuus took
control of the land. The seas
swarmed with jumbo sweatpants
and sensible shoes.
And it was not so good.

It's no secret that pregnancy doth not bring out one's inner glamour girl. Hormones flow, stomachs protrude, and once-clear complexions zigzag with "nonspecific dermatitis." Workouts are traded in for TiVo. A nondescript sack filled with Cheetos replaces the once-chic hobo. And fashion obsessions are usurped by fantasies of tucking into a vat of buttery mac and cheese. Yes, denying one's fashion instincts and reaching for your fat pants—those baggy sweats in your bottom drawer reserved for sitting about the house on Sundays—is a natural response to pregnancy. As a career fashionista (I have served as *Chicago Tribune* style columnist, a trend reporter for NBC, and a style expert for *USA Today* and *Vogue*), I envisioned my pregnancy following in the chic, minimally swollen footsteps of Gwen, Heidi, and Gwyneth. But as the first twelve pounds wrapped themselves around my midsection, I began to cave. The urge to hide in jumbo-sized clothing was over-whelming. I garbed myself in my husband's button-downs. Over sweats. Yoga pants became to-the-office pants. One morning, in my tenth week, I glanced at my dumpy reflection in the mirror as I left for work. In my expansive, dog-walking pantaloons-and-sweatshirt combo, I bore an uncanny resemblance to my potato-picking Russian ancestors. There was no question. **The Baggy Belarus look had to go.**

I hit my local chain maternity store. Nausea washed over me. Where were the sportif strapless dresses and va-va-voom bejeweled shifts worn by the current spate of knocked-up celebs? The pricey drawstring pants (paired

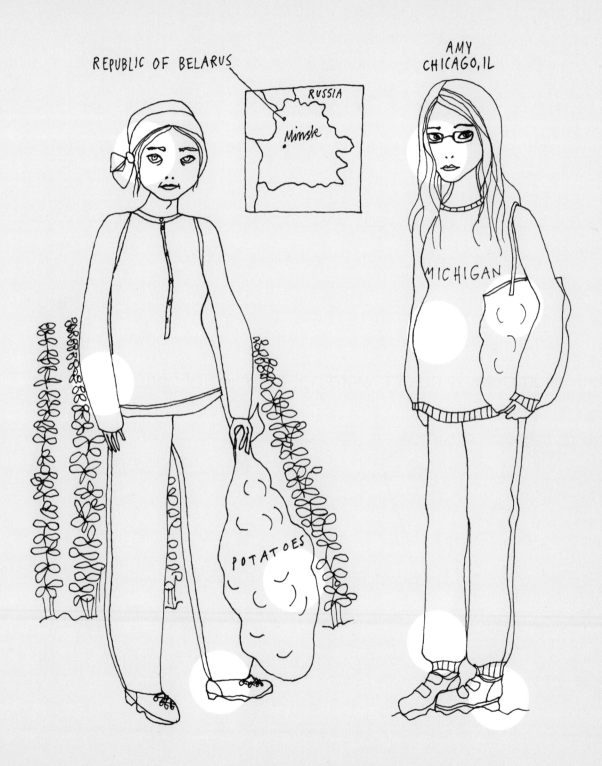

REPUBLIC OF BELARUS

RUSSIA

Minsk

AMY
CHICAGO, IL

MICHIGAN

POTATOES

with ONE HOT MAMA tees), drab button-downs, and decidedly non–Tory Burch tunics were simply not the look that I had in mind. I waddled to Starbucks and pondered my fashion future. I had built a career on style. How could I allow my self-esteem and professional credibility to be eradicated by polyester-blend leisure wear?

Then I had an epiphany: Forget investing my unborn child's college tuition on a full-blown maternity wardrobe. **Bump-savvy celebs were not miracles of nature.** They had simply mastered the high art of mix-and-match fertility fashion, a combination of must-have maternity with easy civilian silhouettes that embraced and enhanced their bump. I might lack Gwyneth's gene code, but a decade of covering fashion shows and interviewing beauty gurus gave me confidence that I, a scrappy five-foot-four editrix, could eschew pregnancy's frump factor and step up to the fashion plate.

I knocked back some Tums and got down to the business of reworking my existing wardrobe. Skinny jeans, skimpy tops, and anything that made me look and feel like five pounds of bologna in a one-pound bag were packed away; empire-waist dresses, tunics, and other bump-friendly silhouettes were positioned front and center. Lycra (from my mom's Jane Fonda days) became my second skin. **Big baubles were my new best friends.** And eye-catching accents—vintage jackets, exotic reptilian bags, capes and shawls, colorful thigh-length sweaters, hardware-laden oversized totes—were my joie de vivre. I cast Pucci-esque innerwear as outerwear, skirts as dresses, and chain belts as necklaces. I revisited seasons-old wrap dresses and off-the-wall knits from storage. **I raided Grandma's closet for Jackie O scarves and quirky accents like Peruvian coin belts and carved jade pendants.** Later, when my bump materialized for the whole world to see, I purchased only core maternity items that could be accessorized for every occasion—a pair of designer pregnancy jeans, a super-long, stretchy black tank top, maternity tights, a chic maternity pencil skirt, and one pair of multitasking black trousers. I bought non-maternity pieces—black bias-cut and empire-waist jersey dresses (cleverly cut to accommodate a bump), a groovy, unstructured sweater/shawl, an early DKNY leather tunic—that would work during my pregnancy and beyond. I borrowed maternity and non-maternity items from friends. I took the fashion credo "God is in the details" to heart and had a blast "super-accessorizing." The key to preggo chic? Creativity. Effort. And the commitment to pushing the sartorial envelope even as you feel your breakfast rising in your throat.

Bump It Up is a cheat sheet to chic, a pregnancy primer that shows moms-to-be how a handful of wardrobe basics can yield dozens of jaw-dropping maternity ensembles. The book's breezy, tip-filled format and fashion cartoons are designed to help you, my pregnant friend, glean, trimester by trimester, style information before "PADD" (pregnancy attention deficit disorder; see Preggo Glossary) kicks in. A checklist system based on three crucial points—the Uniform, Add-ons, and Wow Factor—fine-tunes for pregnancy the editorial concept of garment rotation. **Armed with the basics and a flair for the dramatic, pregnant women can create maximum style with a minimum investment in maternity-specific clothing.**

To visually emphasize this point, I called upon fashion designers such as Nicole Miller, Donna Karan, Milly, Diane von Furstenberg, and Isaac Mizrahi to create original sketches that showcase pregnancy silhouettes that are at once fashionable and functional. We're all obsessed with fashion mags and celebrity tabloids. To get you, dear reader, the most in-the-know tips on the planet, I stepped

behind the scenes of the glossies and canvassed

the real style mavens—designers, editors, publicists, and

socialites—responsible for launching trends among

celebrities and the stylists who assemble them. In "Advice

from the A-list," high-profile beauty and fashion folks

share the experiences that enabled them to finesse the

incredible bulk of pregnancy. And for those who are

served up hormonally induced lumps and bumps instead

of the coveted pregnancy glow, celeb skin gurus weigh

in on how you too can tap into that (faux) radiance.

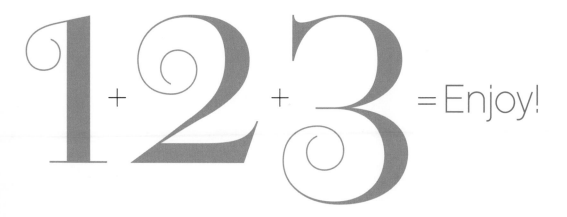

1 + 2 + 3 = Enjoy!

PREGGO GLOSSARY

The moment the double lines of your pregnancy test confirm your bun-in-the-oven status, you are privy to a cornucopia of new vocabulary. Sharing these terms with other moms and moms-to-be is your ticket to an elite members-only club.

BABYMOON: the "last hurrah"-themed vacation usually taken in the seventh month of pregnancy (since flying is not recommended after the seventh month)

BLAST OFF: serious gas released (by you) into the environment—retreat, retreat!

BOOBAGE: showing extreme cleavage

BOYFRIEND JACKET: a longer, slightly structured blazer that features men's tailoring, e.g., lapels

CAKE-AND-BAKE: the tragic phenomenon of a woman who has applied too much bronzer

CAMOUFLAGE CLOTHING: loosely fitting non-maternity garments with flowy fabrics, skillful draping, and generous pleats used to hide trimester 1 poundage

CARB LOADING: the inability to feel well unless consuming Wheat Thins, pretzels, cinnamon-raisin bagels, or coffee cake

CIVILIAN CLOTHING: Non-maternity garments

CONTRACTIVE TOURETTE'S SYNDROME: a temporary condition characterized by uncontrollable cussing during the early stages of labor

DEFCON 4: the secret alert code to husband and friends to find a bathroom ASAP so you can avoid an explosion that will threaten national security

DESPERATION CLOTHING: garments that you would absolutely retch at in a non-pregnant state but that you purchased in a stress-induced state

DOWDIFIER: an item that imparts a frumpy look (e.g., septuagenarian-style loafers, sweatpants, oversized tent shirts)

FAT PANTS: elasticized and oft unattractive pants for days when you feel too huge to squeeze into anything else

FAUX GLOW: artificially induced radiance designed to mimic the sun-kissed luminosity of A-list celebrities (e.g., J. Lo)

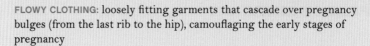

FLOWY CLOTHING: loosely fitting garments that cascade over pregnancy bulges (from the last rib to the hip), camouflaging the early stages of pregnancy

FRUMP PATROL: the once-over you must give yourself in a full-length mirror to eliminate dumpy elements from selected outfit

GARMENT ROTATION: an editorial concept involving skillful rotation of basics with accessories to create dozens of smashing looks

INVESTMENT PIECE: a garment or accessory that you can rationalize spending lots of money on because of its timeless appeal and your faith that it can be worn for decades

LAYERING: the strategic juxtaposition of basic items of clothing and accessories that transform mere garments into a look

LAYETTE: teeny, tiny, to-die-for coming-home-from-the-hospital ensemble for the baby

LBD: the little black dress that works for almost every occasion

MEX HEX: the uncontrollable urge to score enchiladas and guacamole

MUFFIN TOP: The unattractive blubber that hangs over a waistband when pants are too tight and/or tops are too short

"NOW AND LATER": clothing that works both during pregnancy and afterward in your starring role as mom

PADD: pregnancy attention deficit disorder, a temporary affliction that impedes a pregnant woman's ability to focus on activities (except eating) for more than twelve minutes

PREGNANCY BRAIN: forgetfulness that leads to the weekly loss of one's wallet, cell phone, and prescription eyewear

PREGNANCY MASK: hormonally induced dark spots that can form around the mouth and eyes

PUSH PRESENT: that special congratulatory bauble awarded to new moms for providing hubby/partner with his bundle of joy

STRUCTURED CLOTHING: fabulous but non-preggo-friendly clothing featuring a tight fit and sharp tailoring—e.g., nipped-and-tucked jackets, straight-leg trousers, and blazers equipped with linebacker shoulders

SUPER-ACCESSORIZING: editorial term for hard-core layering involving mixing and matching bangles, cocktail rings, oversized tote, and groovy belt into one look

VPL: visible panty lines: a definite no-no

Bloated on the Bias

Nothing frumps you up
like . . . hiding in your husband's
jeans . . . bushy caterpillar
eyebrows . . . unkempt, frizzy
hair . . . no makeup . . . a velour
tracksuit . . . muffin top . . .
college sweatshirts worn any time
other than exercise . . . VPL . . .

You've done it! You're knocked up! Successfully inserted Bun in Oven! Glee. Joy. Exhilaration. Fast-forward to week 3. Double-blue-line delight dissipates as boobs explode into honeydews and belly busts triumphantly beyond restraining waistband. You're nauseous, tired, and flipping out as your carefully cultivated wardrobe begins to resemble Barbie clothing. After a savory midnight snack you wake up in a sweat thinking a *20,000 Leagues Under the Sea*–sized octopus is squeezing the life out of you, but then you realize it's just your nightgown clinging to your bod like Saran Wrap on gooey Brie. You tap your slumbering husband. Emergency lingerie emancipation required.

Keeping mum about your pregnancy during the first three months is beyond frustrating (the risk of miscarriage is reduced after the first trimester). **"I'm not a binge eater— I'm pregnant!"** you want to screech at co-workers whom you imagine are eyeballing your gargantuan rump. But it's only week 4, and save five or so pounds, you look the same, just bloated. **Slyly masking your newfound curves ain't easy.** Your goal? To simply not look fat. So what do you do? How do you assemble yourself during that in-between-bloat-and-belly phase? Instead of heading to a maternity shop in your first trimester, plan on getting through that pre-bump phase with the help of camouflage clothing—loosely fitting non-maternity garments with flowy fabrics, skillful draping, and generous pleats. The right breezy silhouette plus heels and a few accessories will create an illusion of a waist, preventing watercooler snoops from tossing your name into the rumor mill.

CAMOUFLAGE CLOTHING: HOW TO MASK YOUR MOUND TILL WEEK 12

During the first trimester, some women gain fifteen pounds, while others, especially those who suffer from extreme nausea and vomiting, gain almost nothing. At ten weeks, I had ten extra pounds clinging to my formerly petite frame. I remember the frustration clearly. My staple of form-fitting dresses magnified the bloat. Tailored button-downs made me look like a Budweiser-loving Buddha. Slim-cut trousers became a boa constrictor sucking the life from me. Whatever your body size or shape, there is only one thing to do when you feel fat and dumpy. Take the focus away from the midsection and elongate your silhouette. The trick? A bit of sartorial sleight of hand.

Trade in structured, tight, and tailored tops and dresses for loose-fitting pieces that drape and flow over the belly and hips. Pay attention to proportion. If it's baggy on top, it has to be fitted on the bottom. Keep skirt and dress lengths at or just above the knee to play up your legs. And to get you out of the preggo dumps, always wear a heel. I am not talking *Sex and the City* spikes. A kitten heel, a wedge, or a boot with a mid-range heel will elongate your frame. Chances are, you already own some flowy tops (loose-fitting fabric that covers the area from the last rib to the hip) and dresses that will work as pre-maternity wear. And if you don't, buy a few breezy "now and later" garments to wear now and after the baby is born. Be open-minded. It's critical to accept that, though your brain wants to toss on form-fitting clothing, your belly and butt are vehemently opposed. Listen to your body and go flowy.

camouflage clothing

\ (ˈka-mə-fläzh ˈklō-thiŋ) \ *n.* \ breezy non-maternity garments that cleverly mask pregnancy poundage.

HOT TIP
Every fashion editor who was interviewed for this book concurred that heels visually lengthen the legs, elongate the silhouette, and offer a literal lift from that dowdy, bloated feeling.

Get high!
Best bets to lengthen the silhouette

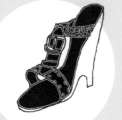

HEDGE ON THE WEDGE: The wedge heel offers height and support and is much easier to wear than a wobbly stiletto. Wedges balance thicker ankles and calves and are available for every season and in every heel height.

HERE, KITTY, KITTY: Popularized by Audrey Hepburn, this slender micro heel (about 1¼ to 2 inches) looks great with everything. A mule is a backless kitten heel.

GET THE BOOT: For fall and winter pregnancies, boots are essential. Ankle boots with a chunky heel and slightly pointed toe add height to jeans and trousers. When wearing a dress, a fitted to-the-knee boot is slimming and lengthening. Calf-length or ankle boots are okay with a dress if your legs are thin. Avoid them if you have thicker legs because this height makes legs look heavier. If you're on the tall side, a slouchy to-the-knee flat boot can be worn with jeans. Cowboy boots are the ultimate pregnancy footwear. They have major support and enough of a heel to elongate your legs.

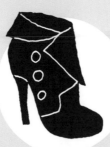

REWORK YOUR CLOSET:
WHAT TO USE, WHAT TO LOSE

A snapshot of your changing body: Flat is becoming full.
Straight is going curvy. And, though you fantasize about
reaching in and retrieving a flattering outfit, your closet's
current incarnation is not equipped to handle your voluptified
figure. Face it. It's time for some wardrobe nip/tuck.

　　Approach your closet with a pregnancy mindset and
start organizing. Don't get depressed by that form-fitting
dress. Pack it, along with skinny jeans and any other
clothing that resembles a second skin, all away. Structured
garments—sharply tailored skirts and trousers, austere
nipped-at-the-waist blazers, and jackets with linebacker
shoulders—are restrictive in trimester 1 and unwearable by
month 6. And sorry, biker babes. Leather and pregnancy are
like foie gras and ketchup—a freakish combo. What to keep?
Garments that naturally play down the waist and emphasize
legs, arms, and bust. Think relaxed fit. Drapey, flowy,
ethereal. Dresses—wrap, shift, empire-waist, and trapeze
(see pages 11–12)—are ideal, as they disguise bottom
heaviness. Long tanks and to-the-hip tunics (see p. 10)
cover a bulging midsection. Jeans and trousers with a lower,
nonbinding waistband can often be worn until the second
trimester (see "Five Fast Fertility Fixes," page 9). Soft silhouettes offer pitch-perfect pregnancy panache. Examples?
Unstructured jackets, thin, open-at–the-front cashmere
knits, soft, thigh-length tops with interesting details like a
kimono sleeve. And magical maneuvers can be performed
upon black skirts with a stretchy waistband. Examine pieces
in storage. Your burgeoning bump may give new meaning
to last season's dress. Accessorizing is that extra step that
will take an outfit from blah to baroque. Silky scarves and
the oft-mocked pashmina can be looped nonchalantly around

structured clothing

\ (ˈstrək-chərd ˈklō-thiŋ) \ n. \
sharply tailored, fitted
garments favored by power-
dressing execs and
hard-edged Victoria
Beckham types.

the neck to add color and Parisienne chic. Belts—thick and thin—will become useful to wear above and below the belly in the second trimester. Larger bags are must-haves to use as a physical shield in trimester 1 and balance out your proportion when your belly explodes in the forthcoming weeks. And jewelry—the bigger the better—should be positioned smack in the middle of your dresser to work into every look. Trust me, a pared-down closet is an efficient closet.

Bottoms Up! Extend the Life of Your Civilian Clothes

While you're going flowy on top, pants and trousers still pose a problem. Caught in that precarious in-between-bump-and-bloat phase, you find that nothing quite fits, yet you're not ready (rightly so!) to take the plunge into maternity. Though I had gained about ten pounds in my first trimester, I could still shoehorn myself into existing jeans, skirts, and trousers, since my legs and butt were roughly the same size. The problem was with the button. Two freshly minted handfuls of flesh prohibited closure of my pants. What, I mused, could enable me to wear my jeans and trousers with the button splayed comfortably open?

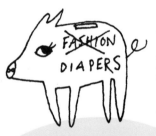

HOT TIP

Pregnancy is the perfect time to streamline your wardrobe—and make some cash. While you're packing away non-pregnancy-appropriate garb, gather the decades-old pieces—the goatskin unitard, June Cleaver chiffon dresses, thigh-high boots, leather trench coat—that no longer jibe with your current look. March these items over to your local consignment store or sell them on eBay to start your diaper fund.

Five Fast Fertility Fixes

1. When your jeans or trousers still fit everywhere except the belly, a **SIMPLE RUBBER BAND** can offer additional breathing room. Leave jeans unfastened and loop the rubber band around the button and buttonhole. This sartorial trickery is easily concealed with a hip-length T-shirt, some sassy, dangly scarves, or a cute scarf worn as a wide kimono belt.

2. Two weeks later, when the notion of zipping your pants becomes comical, it's time for the elasticized **BELLY BAND**. This soft, seamless, stretchy band is a respirator for civilian pants and skirts. By miraculously sheathing unzipped, rolled-to-the-hips pants, the belly band extends the life span of jeans and trousers. Too-tight skirts can still be worn by pushing the waistband below the hip and covering the bulging fabric with the band. Again, a lightweight, thigh-length top romantically draped over the band camouflages your handiwork. You can buy the bands at most maternity stores, or online (try www.ingridandisabel.com), or you can make your own with store-bought dance-wear fabric.

3. A more polished approach to resizing your trousers? Have your tailor sew into the side seams **SMALL TRIANGULAR ELASTIC BANDS** that can be removed post-baby.

4. **CONTROL-TOP UNDIES** like Flexees or Soma help to fit distended bodies into pants, dresses, and skirts. *Switch to maternity-specific undies by month 4.*

5. A **BODY SLIMMER** like those made by Maidenform, Donna Karan's Body Perfect collection, or Spanx slims out thighs and chisels the waistline during the first trimester. With thick-gage Lycra extending from below the boobs to the ankles, Spanx High-Falutin' Footless Pantyhose is a trimester 1 fan favorite. There is even a thoughtful crotch opening to make life easier when Mother Nature calls. You can also switch to maternity-specific slimmers in the second trimester.

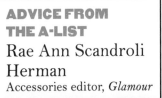

ADVICE FROM THE A-LIST

Rae Ann Scandroli Herman
Accessories editor, *Glamour*

The first three months of pregnancy are the hardest because you feel thick. Try to wear fuller (non-maternity) dresses for as long as possible. I would rather stretch out my regular clothing and not spend the money on maternity wear until I really need it. Later, after giving birth [Rae Ann speaks from experience—she was pregnant with *bébé* number three when I interviewed her!], you can always belt or tailor the stretched-out dress or shirt.

SPECTACULARLY SLIMMING SILHOUETTES FOR TRIMESTER UNO

On the subject of camouflage clothing, there are certain shapes renowned for their ability to disguise bottom heaviness. The sexy, unstructured shapes of the sixties—think boho Kate Hudson meets Jackie Kennedy in Swinging London—offer major style (and coverage) in all the right places. Here's my advice: If you are already a fan of these iconic styles, wear them with renewed appreciation. If not, this is the time to become one. Sound investment pieces (see Preggo Glossary) and easy to wear, those non-maternity silhouettes will not expire at the nine-month mark. In fact, if you don't muck them up with guacamole during your pregnancy, they will still look smashing as office garb/out-on-the-town gear long after the baby is born. Where to go? Designer resale shops, sample sales, eBay, and websites that offer vintage clothing such as Decadesinc.com (see Resources) are all good options. Stunning clothing and accessories can be had at bargain-basement prices. Why? Models, actresses, and your average shopaholic consign new and gently used clothing the moment the next big thing emerges. I bought tons of Marc Jacobs and Chanel at Decades in Los Angeles for one-third the retail price!

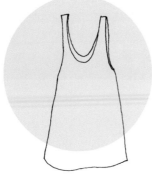

←Talk Tunic to Me

The breezy dress-me-up, dress-me-down tunic gets an A+ in masking girth. Popularized by such style luminaries as Babe Paley and Talitha Getty, this versatile thigh-length style is beloved for its ability to showcase boobage and hide bloatage. Embellished silk tunics (think Barbra Streisand in Scaasi for her *Funny Girl* Oscar win) are divine for a night out. Go casual with soft, colorful cotton tunics over slim-fitting jeans or capris. A silky empire-waist tunic with jeans and a shawl can go to an of-the-moment eatery with heels or to a July 4 barbecue. Layering accessories—necklaces, bangles, and rings—pack style punch into a simple look. *The tunic may not be the best option for a pear shape. It can break at the hip and magnify bottom heaviness.*

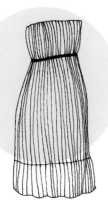

←Build Your Empire

Start your love affair with the empire waist. This genius silhouette gathers under the breast and falls loosely to the hip, knee, or floor, covering bulging bellies and butts with cascading fabric. The empire waist also puts the focus on the arms and shoulders, places where pregnancy weight does not manifest itself.

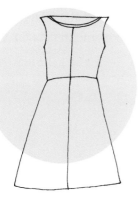

←Meet the A-Line

Another concealer extraordinaire is the classic A-line dress. Narrow on the top, flaring at the hemline, this garment is designed to graze the midsection and makes one's gams the focal point. Worn with heels and a smart jacket, the above-the-knee A-line is perfect for the office or a cocktail party. For winter, just toss on a cardigan and tights.

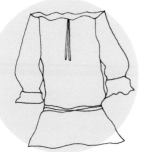

←Bask in the Blouson

Billowy fabric blouses over a fitted waistband (which acts as a girdle) to cover the growing belly. Wear with jeans, trousers, or a skirt. Very *Charlie's Angels*.

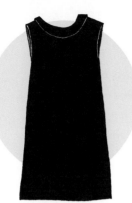

←Seismic Shift

Channel Gidget. Or my preggo icon, Gwen Stefani, with the flirty old-school shift. Cut straight from the shoulders and flowing away from the hips, this above-the-knee dress is easy to wear and disguises thickening thighs and other forms of bottom heaviness. Season after season, this shape is reinterpreted and can be found at retailers from Target to Nordstrom.

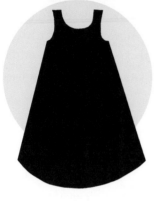

←Trapeze Artist

With a more pronounced flare (à la trapezoid) from the hips, the breezy trapeze dress took the fashion world by storm when trotted down the YSL catwalk in the 1960s.

These days, fashion folk still clamor for the fit-and-flare shape in the form of dress, trench, and shirt. Dress the trapeze up with heels and jewelry or down with flats for a comfily chic look.

Don't do it!
Sweatpants

Every pregnant woman dreads a favorite pair of jeans becoming too tight to fasten. That awkward feeling leads to slipping into the ultimate comfort clothing: sweatpants. Here's the problem. Sweats are so comfortable, so nonbinding, that you, like the elderly mall rats of Boca Raton, will never want to take them off. To a pregnant woman, sweats are evil. Verboten. The ultimate dowdifier (see Preggo Glossary). Sweats are voluminous, making even the slimmest thighs resemble tree trunks. Sweats make five pounds look like fifteen. They make your butt balloon. They inspire waddling. You want to wear them at home? Fine. But they erode your glam appeal by 1,000 percent and, when worn in public, will make you feel like an elephant amongst gazelles.

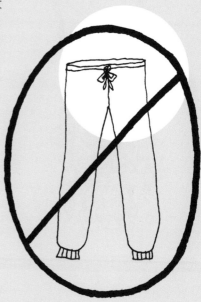

GO FOR THE GOLD: ELEVATE BASICS WITH A DASH OF FLASH

Once you are in possession of key pieces of camouflage clothing, elevate the flowy tops and basic silhouettes by working in a dash of flash with gold accessories. When you think about some of your favorite perennially chic celebs peeping out from the pages of *People* magazine, you will notice a trend: shots of gold in the form of jewelry, belts, and bags. This is nothing new. Screen sirens from the forties jazzed up their black column gowns and midnight-blue "New Look" Dior suits with stunning gold jewelry. The mod sixties hiked up hemlines and incorporated gold for maximum counterculture effect. The seventies ushered in Farrah Fawcett and the disco era with va-va-voom chain belts and drippy gold earrings accenting matchy knit ensembles and the Candie's spike heels. The eighties = Studio 54, an homage to flash and cash. My point? Gold accessories, real or faux, have an edge. They add of-the-moment oomph and polish to basics. The look reads "I am—and will remain post-childbirth—a hot mama!"

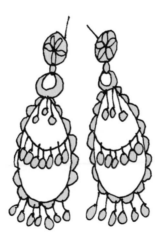

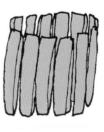

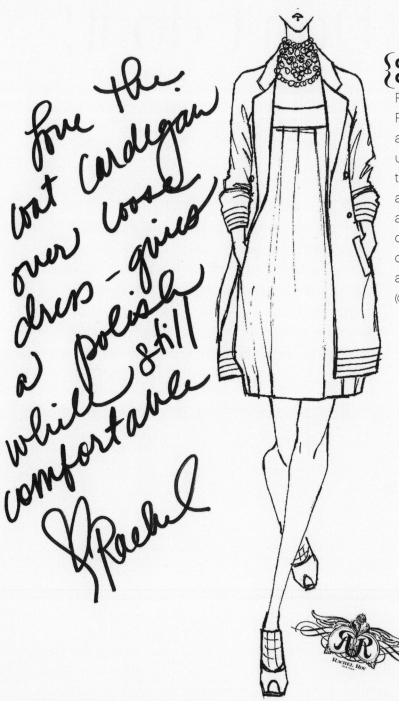

*love the
coat cardigan
over loose
dress – gives
a polish
while still
comfortable*

Rachel

Don't do it!
Lycra in Trimester 1

Visions of bump-hugging dresses will dance in your head. Ignore them. At this point, you have a bulge, not a bump. Many think that Lycra and other skin-tight fabrics will function as a girdle, sucking in their padded rump and stomach. With the equivalent of a dozen bagels in your belly, clingy fabrics will accent the negative, delivering a freakish muffin-top homage to Britney Spears post-meltdown. Remember: Trimester 1 is all about camouflage. When you feel the lure of microfiber, peer into the mirror and chant this phrase aloud three times: "Drape and flow are what I need now; Lycra will make me look like a cow." Fret not, in a few weeks your shining Lycra moment will arrive.

TRIMESTER 1 POP QUIZ: BODY LANGUAGE 101

Nearly all women feel overwhelmed by weight gain. Set the tone for your day by denying the urge to hide in your fat pants (see Preggo Glossary). Pulling yourself together is the key ingredient of looking and feeling great during pregnancy. The proof is in the triple-chocolate fudge pudding. Try this little exercise on for size:

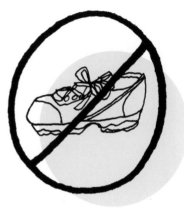

Lesson 1: Train Wreck à la Mode

You wake up and dress to reflect your emotions: sweatpants, sneakers, and your comfy college sweatshirt. Then, without so much as glancing in the mirror, you run out to do some errands . . . How does your dumpy demeanor impact your body language?

A Do you saunter sexily down the catwalk of life, head held high, like Giselle Bündchen?

B Do your feet drag? Do your shoulders sag? Would you rather crawl back into bed with a dozen Krispy Kreme doughnuts than get dressed and face the day?

C Do you look up in surprise when someone in the supermarket asks if you are available to clean her house next week because her cleaning lady is on vacation?

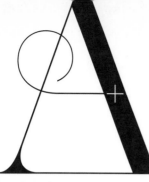

Lesson 2: Going Glam

You feel like Roseanne but are determined to channel Anne
Hathaway. Wear a flattering, loose, belted black dress, fun
earrings, and some glamifying mascara and lipstick. Add
some height and a soupçon of glamour with a pair of mid-
range heels. Pop on some cute sunglasses, and out you go.
How does your pulled-together, well-proportioned look
impact your body language?

A Is your gait light and airy—like a member of the plus-size
division of Elite Models?

B Do you feel upbeat and attractive—like yourself, but
bloated?

C Is your budding belly but a minor detail of your show-
stopping look?

D All of the above.

Lesson 3: Effortless Elán

Deny your inner hausfrau and put some effort into your
appearance. Contain your bloat with control-top undies and
wriggle into your almost-too-snug jeans. Layer a breezy
tank with a jangle of pendants and a gauzy Stevie Nicks–
style scarf. Add heels and a giant clutch bag.

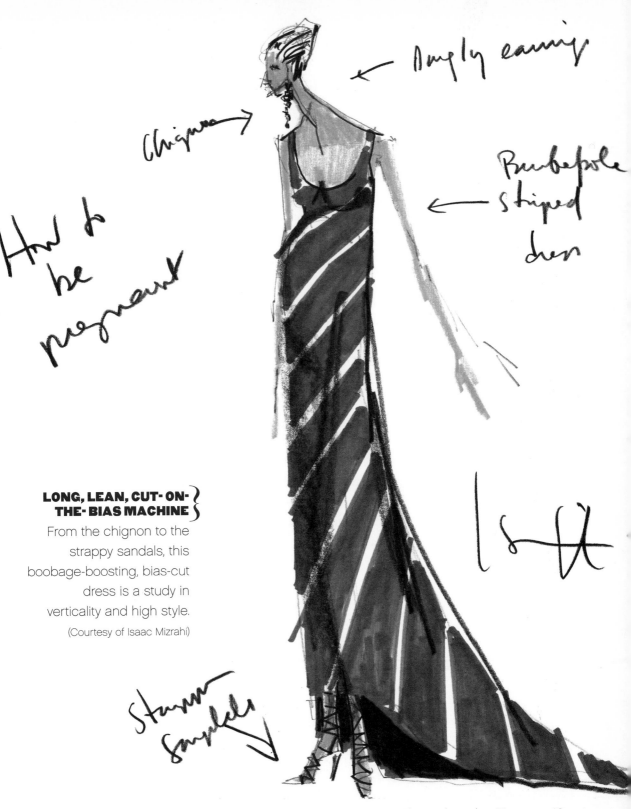

Amply earring

Chignon

Burbepole striped dress

How to be pregnant

LONG, LEAN, CUT- ON- THE- BIAS MACHINE
From the chignon to the strappy sandals, this boobage-boosting, bias-cut dress is a study in verticality and high style.
(Courtesy of Isaac Mizrahi)

Strappy Sandals

seasonless dressing

\ ('sē-z°n-ləs 'dre-siŋ) \ *n.* \ skillful layering of lightweight summer basics for year-round style.

RETHINK YOUR SUMMER WARDROBE: THE JOYS OF SEASONLESS DRESSING

While you're editing your closet, examine some of your favorite magazines. See that model in *Glamour* wearing a cute gauzy camisole under a slim-cut wool blazer? A billowy silk dress paired with a cable-knit sweater and ankle boots in *Lucky*? Thanks to the fashion industry's love affair with layering, a huge trend has emerged: seasonless dressing. Nylon neutrals in January! Sleeveless print dresses in March! Silky summer fabrics and nubby knits are living harmoniously on and off the runway. How does this relate to the soon-to-be mama? In pregnancy, as in so many areas of life, the grass seems oh-so-much greener on the other side. Summer pregnancies seem easier because they're all about breezy, easy dresses and comfy sandals. But the heat causes increased swelling. Winter pregnancies give you free license to cocoon in mountains of wool. But the weight of extra fabric adds pounds to an already exaggerated frame. The airy tops and dresses previously only trotted out for lazy summer days are the building blocks of year-round fashion. You can make use of existing summer staples for a winter pregnancy and know that roomy non-maternity pregnancy purchases—the black silk shift, the brown jersey wrap dress, the sleeveless silky bias-cut tunic—are solid "now and later" (see Preggo Glossary) investment pieces that will be amortized throughout the years by adding tights, a belt, and boots. Underscoring the sensibility of this layering trend for pregnantistas, Donna Karan recently designed a maternity capsule collection based on—you guessed it—seasonless basics. Seasonless dressing will change your life—and save you money.

Six Ways to Winterize
Your Spring/Summer Clothing

1. A silky slip dress is a year-round basic. Add boots, tights, and a **ROOMY KNIT** (can be belted).

2. **JERSEY** is a seasonless fabric in any permutation.

3. Gauzy and whisper-thin **CASHMERE TANK TOPS** are sporty, easy wardrobe staples.

4. Sleeveless black or brown tank and T-shirt dresses can be paired with a **BOYFRIEND JACKET** (see Preggo Glossary) or grandpa knit.

5. Add **TIGHTS** and **BOOTS** to a cotton shirtdress or sundress for a great fall look.

6. A strapless knee-length empire waist or a black maxidress can be paired with a **SHRUG** or **CARDIGAN** for a smashing fall/winter look.

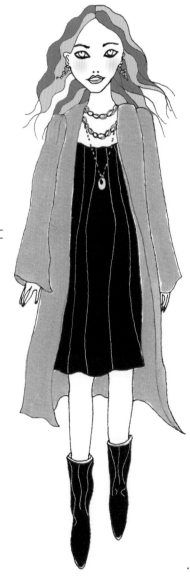

BRIGHT YOUNG THING

GO WITH THE FLOW }

Here DKNY features a versatile maternity look based on a seasonless empire-waist ruffled tunic. For summer, the silky fit-and-flare tunic is worn with leggings and heels. For winter, the very same tunic can be paired with a cashmere shrug and to-the-knee boots. NOTE: The low-cut top and empire waist put the focus on the arms and chest. The flowy tunic is countered with tight leggings. Heels elongate the whole look. (Courtesy of DKNY)

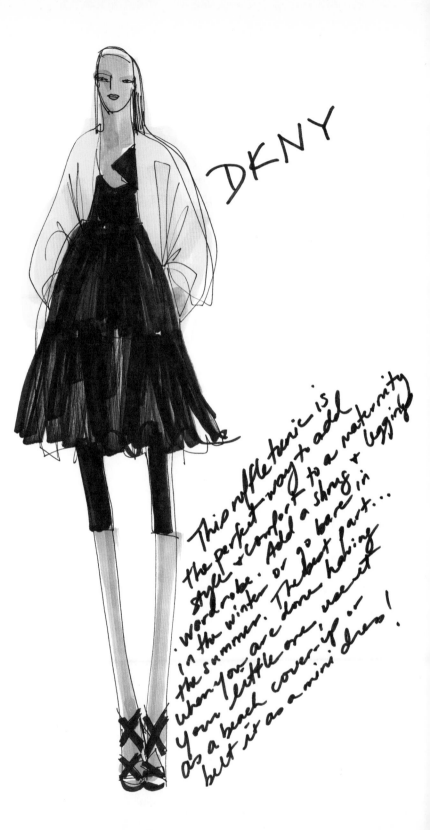

DKNY

This ruffle tunic is the perfect way to add style & comfort to a maternity wardrobe. Add a shrug in the winter or go bare in the summer. The best part... when you are done having your little one, use it as a beach cover-up or belt it as a mini dress!

Layering 101

Plain pasta is okay. But when you layer it with sausage, mozzarella, peas, and a zippy cream sauce, you've got a savory meal. The same notion applies to style. Layering, the juxtaposition of fabrics, textures, hemlines, and accessories, is the Holy Grail of fashion folk. Whether you are pregnant or not, the confluence of style elements is what transforms random combinations of garments into a Look. Check this out: Pregnancy jeans with a black chiffon tank top is fade-into-the-woodwork nice. But mix in glitzy kitten-heel slides, a Pucci-esque swingy trapeze jacket, a heavy gold pendant, gold earrings, and some fun bangles, and you've made a statement. The point? Because your accessories are so dramatic, you can rework that fade-into-the-woodwork chiffon top and jeans a dozen different ways and nobody will figure out that you're actually wearing the same "uniform" day in and day out. Layering, a critical element at every stage of pregnancy dressing, allows the savvy pregnantista to invest in a small quantity of quality basics and effectively "bump them up" into a look. In fashion, God is most definitely in the details . . . or, rather, the accessories.

layering
\ ('lā-y°r-iŋ) \ n. \
an editorial technique; the combination of textures, hemlines, and accessories that takes a basic outfit from blah to baroque.

Hot Flash 101

Layering serves a physical purpose as well as a fashion goal: protection from estrogen-singed hot flashes. Sky-high hormone levels are the science behind the phrase "bun in the oven." I almost passed out when my first hot flash occurred. It was December and I was out to lunch in a black form-fitting turtleneck. Suddenly I became flushed and rivulets of sweat began dripping from my hairline into my Cobb salad (extra bacon, cheese, and avocado). I swiftly made my way to the bathroom, ripped off my sweater, and doused myself in cold water. From that point on, *turtleneck* was a synonym for *torture*. I became a seasonless-dressing fanatic, layering open sweaters and jackets with silky sleeveless tunics or dresses. Fair warning, cashmere lovers. Be prepared, so that when your inner thermometer swings from polar to tropical in twelve seconds flat, you are not trapped inside a luxury straitjacket.

THE LOOK: PULLING IT ALL TOGETHER—CAMOUFLAGE, PROPORTION, AND LONG, LEAN LINES

Once you've identified the four or five silhouettes that work for you, getting dressed will be a breeze. Again, the trick is to mix and match dynamic accessories with body-skimming garments that strategically ebb and flow over the belly. Select "camouflage" garments that create long, lean lines in order to play down the waist and emphasize legs, bust, and arms. Amp up your basics with gold bangles, tribal beads, cocktail rings, exotic belts, or whatever interesting accent pieces you have on hand. Bring the focal point up to your face, neck, and arms with earrings, lower-cut tops, and dresses that display décolletage. Pull it all together with a great bag and shoes.

a look

\ (ā 'lů k) \ *n.* \ the successful pairing, or layering, of various fashion elements that together transform individual pieces of clothing into a style statement.

WEEKEND WARRIOR

ELONGATE THE SILHOUETTE
A dangly scarf creates verticality and hides the belly.

PROPORTION AND LAYERING
Add a few long necklaces—gold, beads, pendants—to rein in baggy tops and lend an element of style.

FERTILITY FIX
Wearing a high-waisted body slimmer under pants, skirts, or dresses will minimize midriff, thighs, and rear.

MAKE A FOCAL POINT
Use accessories to draw attention away from your belly and add polish to the look.

CAMOUFLAGE
Longer-to-the-hip tunics are functional because they drape over the pants button, which is held together by a rubber band.

PROPORTION
Pair roomy tops with trousers or jeans that are more tailored or slim-cut.

STREAMLINE
Heels—even a slight kitten heel—elongate the body and reduce that "I feel like a stout hunk of lard" feeling.

A Few More Pulling-It-All-Together Pointers

1. Add shape to amorphous garments with a belt. You can use a wide belt at the hips so fabric can be bloused over a bulging belly. Or use an elasticized belt below the bust to create an empire silhouette.

2. The empire waist accentuates the rib cage, giving the wearer an attenuated frame. An elevated just-under-the-bust waistline offers your tummy a full range of bloatdom.

3. If you have gained first-trimester weight in your butt, a black sleeveless shift or A-line dress is a chic place to hide. This essential masks bottom heaviness and can be effortlessly accessorized.

4. A shawl creates verticality and camouflages as it drapes elegantly over the midsection.

5. Wear V-necks, tanks, and lower-cut tops, which focus on your arms and shoulders, where pregnancy weight does not manifest itself.

HOT TIP
Scarves, whether lightweight cotton or heavy cashmere, are the ultimate layering piece. Aside from adding color and contrast, a flowing scarf at the belly covers your bulge from the world.

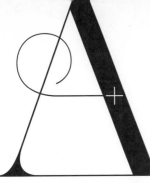

PREGNANT? SHRIIIEEEKK!!! WHAT WILL YOU WEAR???!

Pregnancy used to translate into the fashion doldrums for nine months or so. Not anymore. Pregnancy allows you to discover a new style. Confronted with a new body, for which old proven styles no longer work, one is forced to experiment with new shapes, colors, styles. I never fancied empire waists, but during my pregnancy they were my best friends. Tight, stretchy tops are usually absolutely not my cup of tea, but during pregnancy I wanted to show the world my fabulous little belly—and those huge twins! I don't know if it's the hormones that change one's perspective or if the physical changes really do require adjustments . . . My pregnancy uniforms were form-fitting tops and skirts, empire-waist dresses, and very flowy dresses. At five feet eleven, I have always been able to afford the luxury of flats. The baby belly changed it all. I needed some more height to balance the bump out and look longer and leaner. I rediscovered the sexiness of heels. Pregnancy was a time when I really felt I had to flaunt the femme fatale in me. Heels, clutches, and all those fabulous accessories were my dearest companions.

Morphing into the Queen of Camouflage

DO

* Wear **HEELS**: Stacked, kitten, or wedge heels add a glam edge to any look.
* Consider wearing some of your husband's pin-striped (vertical stripes are slimming) **BUTTON-DOWNS** with fab necklaces and leggings.
* Partner **TO-THE-KNEE BLACK BOOTS** with heels with dresses and skirts to elongate the body.
* Wear only **BLACK OPAQUE TIGHTS** to elongate the body.
* Use **COLORFUL SCARVES** as Japanese-style sashes to cover your unbuttoned non-maternity jeans.
* Always wear **JEWELRY**.
* Prepare for hot flashes by layering **TANK TOPS** under sweaters and jackets.

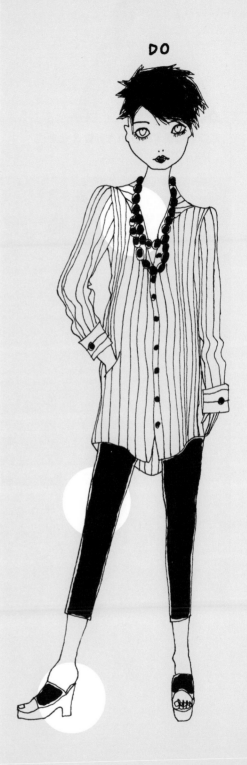

DO

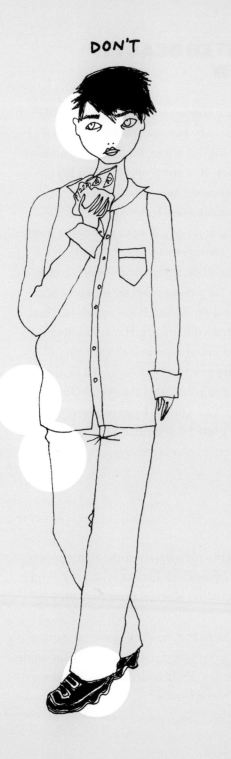

DON'T

* Sport **CLINGY FABRICS** until you have a shapely bump (usually at week 19).
* Wear **OVERSIZED** button-downs with oversized pants.
* Wear shlubby **TRACKSUITS**.
* Wear **NUDE PANTYHOSE**.
* Invest in **MATERNITY CLOTHING** (until the second trimester).
* **FORGET TO TWEEZE** your brows each week. Prenatal vitamins make hair sprout like grass.
* Wear **SNEAKERS** unless you are headed to the gym.

FIRST-TRIMESTER BEAUTY: GET THAT GLOW

Some pregnant women are blessed with that goddess-like glow from within. Not me. My face was peppered with a smorgasbord of dermatological atrocities from the moment I learned of my pregnancy. Red spots appeared on my cheeks. Water retention caused Samsonite-sized luggage to take up residence under my eyes. Itchy eczema patches came and went on my face and body. I went through a bout of acne that would put a teenager's volcanic complexion to shame. I reached out to all of my favorite beauty gurus for help. L.A.–based skin fairy Sonya Dakar (on speed dial from my cell phone) guided me through the rough patches. Literally. Celeb derm extraordinaire Dr. Harold Lancer taught me about melasma prevention and the benefits of microdermabrasion during pregnancy. I surveyed in-the-know moms about home remedies. And thanks to Giorgio Armani's makeup master, Tim Quinn, I learned how to fake that coveted preggo glow by artfully blending mineral-powder foundations, shimmer, and bronzer.

faux glow

\ (fō glō) \ n. \ an artificially induced sun-kissed visage designed to mimic the natural radiance of Bo Derek in *10*, James Bond beauty Ursula Andress, Gisele Bündchen, or Halle Berry.

SKIN CARE: THE ANATOMY OF A GREAT COMPLEXION

Great skin requires a quality skin-care regime that encourages cellular turnover: frequent exfoliation, hydration, and sunscreen application. But what worked pre-pregnancy may not work now.

Evaluate your products and avoid the host of contra-indicated ingredients for pregnancy. Avoid topical kojic acid; vitamin A; retinoids; glycolic, alpha hydroxyl, beta hydroxyl, and salicylic acids; and hydroquinone.

These ingredients can enter your bloodstream and harm the fetus. Synthetic preservatives are a concern since the baby ingests everything that enters your bloodstream. Whether you are a product junkie or a do-it-yourself gal, the "Best Bets" sections later offer of-the-moment skin-care options to get you glowing.

Hydration: "Plump" Juicy Skin, or, the Jessica Alba Effect

Dry skin = haggard face. With a growing fetus literally sucking life from you, your skin will become dehydrated easily. In selecting a cleanser, gentle is the name of the game. Many women are convinced that a high lather is required to remove makeup and cleanse the skin. Actually, suds are created by sodium lauryl sulfate (SLS, an inexpensive foaming agent also found in dishwasher detergent and other household cleansers), which strips oil from the skin, often leaving dry, itchy patches of dermatitis in its wake. Many dermatologists green-light products such as Cetaphil, which contains sodium laureth sulfate (SLES), a far-less-irritating derivative of SLS. Non-lathering cleansing milk (available at every price point from top-tier department stores to Wal-Mart) is a gentle alternative that cleanses without stripping essential oils from the skin.

To moisturize, your skin will need more than a basic lotion. Here's the reality: The baby takes *your* moisture-boosting omega-3 and omega-6 essential fatty acids to develop her little brain, so to stay hydrated, you must replenish. Again. And again. Being pregnant during a Chicago winter (twice) gave me the splendid opportunity to test-drive every moisturizer known to woman. My usual suspects had left me high and dry, so I layered nourishing ingredients like omega-3s, omega-6es, peptides, rose oil, propolis, colostrum serum, aloe vera, and vitamin E in the form of product "cocktails." These ingredients increase water content in the epidermis, a requirement for moist, supple skin. For the really rough red patches on my face and body, I slathered on cult classic Egyptian Magic, an inexpensive cure-all emollient containing beeswax, olive oil, and bee propolis that can be found at Whole Foods. To reduce that dry, cakey feeling midday, pat moisturizer or face oil over your makeup. And drink double the amount of water that you would normally consume. The result is a moist, juicy, "plump" complexion à la Jessica Alba.

BEST BETS: HYDRATION Jurlique Rosewater Balancing Mist or Epicuren Colostrum Hydrating Mist (under and over makeup), Sonya Dakar Omega-3 Repair Complex and Hydrasoft Cream, SkinCeuticals Hydrating B5 Gel, Kate Somerville Quench Hydrating Serum and Deep Tissue Repair, Burt's Bees Radiance Day Lotion, Egyptian Magic Skin Cream, Vanicream Moisturizing Skin Cream.

DIY: HYDRATION Olive oil, sunflower oil, honey, and avocado oil are natural humectants and can be used like a mask. Slick your hair back under a headband and slather one of these oils or honey on your face for ten minutes, then remove with a lather-free cleanser.

Exfoliation: Treat Your Face Like an Heirloom

What happens to Granny's heirloom silver tray when you leave it sitting on the bar too long? It becomes dull and tarnished. Skin is like silver. It gleams when it's polished regularly. Debris, or dead-skin-cell buildup at the surface of the skin, inhibits product penetration and makes your skin lackluster. Sloughing off the dead epidermal cells removes debris and exposes the fresh, living cells that account for bright, healthy-looking skin. For pregnant women, exfoliation is a preventative measure to ward off the dreaded "pregnancy mask," or melasma (for more details, see p. 34). Dr. Harold Lancer, the go-to derm in Beverly Hills (patients include Angie Harmon and Lisa Rinna) for West Coast women on the verge of hormonal meltdowns, is aggressive about putting pregnant patients on a preventative regimen before problems develop. Dr. Lancer believes that aside from avoiding the sun religiously, polishing the skin with professional microdermabrasion is the key to minimizing melasma. "Buffing and toning the skin on the face, neck, and chest with micro-fine crystals at the speed of sound sloughs off the top layer of skin and promotes high cell turnover," he says. Professional microdermabrasion is effective, but you don't need to spend the big bucks for results. There are dozens of mild exfoliants that can do the trick. Look for enzyme-based (papaya, citrus, pineapple, pumpkin, or lactic acid) scrubs with noninvasive granules (stay away from products that contain nuts, as they can cut the skin).

BEST BETS: EXFOLIATION For dry and/or sensitive skin, try Sonya Dakar Enzyme Peeling Cream, Kate Somerville Micro Lactic Polisher, or Pangea Organics Facial Mask. For normal and oily skin, Olay Regenerist Detoxifying Pore Scrub and Epicuren Extra Fine Citrus Herbal Scrub offer the perfect polish.

DIY: EXFOLIATION Mix equal parts yogurt and organic oats into a smooth paste (about ½ cup) and apply to face, neck, and décolletage twice a week.

ADVICE FROM THE A-LIST

Dr. Lisa Airan
New York City's derm du jour

Aside from examining ingredients and being vigilant about sunscreen application, be aware that a host of rashes, some more dangerous than others, can occur throughout pregnancy. If serious eczema or a new skin condition occurs, be safe and see a dermatologist; do not self-diagnose.

Melasma: Beware the Glare

Hormone surges + sun = hideous dark patches called melasma, a.k.a. "pregnancy mask." More than 50 percent of pregnant women develop the darkening of pigmentation around the mouth, cheeks, and forehead also known as hyperpigmentation. How to avoid it? Derms and other skin-care experts concur that, whatever the season, hyper-application of sunblock is imperative. Sun exposure—even when driving in a car or sitting with an open shade on an airplane—can darken existing freckles or stimulate hyperpigmentation. Here's the tongue-twisting explanation: Elevated levels of estrogen and progesterone trigger pigment-producing cells in the skin called melanocytes. The sun's ultraviolet rays cause melanocytes to produce melanin, which causes melasma in a matter of minutes. Dr. Lisa Airan, Manhattan-based skin guru, is known for her cutting-edge approach to pregnancy-induced skin problems. "Sunblock," Airan insists, "is required (all year round) whenever a pregnant woman walks out the door." You can take other measures to avoid melasma. Products containing vitamin C in the form of L-ascorbic acid can control melanin production and inhibit melasma.

HOT TIP
During the spring and summer months, protect your skin from the sun's harmful rays by channeling Sophia Loren with a wide-brimmed sun hat.

Dark, Puffy Eyes: Pack Your Bags

Sadly, exhaustion and poor circulation during pregnancy often invite dark bags under the eyes. An eye cream or serum with ingredients such as elastin, oxygen, collagen, and vitamin E will hydrate your skin and reduce swelling. And in the same way a cup of joe gets you going in the morning, eye creams containing caffeine jump-start circulation, and draw out the excess fluid that causes swelling and dark circles.

BEST BETS: UNDER-EYE BAGS Olay's Regenerist Eye Serum, Weleda Wild Rose Intensive Eye Cream, Dr. Lancer Eye Brightener/Lightener, and Decléor Hydra Flora Hydrating Eye Contour Gel have soothing florals and caffeine to smooth and soothe tired eyes.

DIY: BYE-BYE, BAGS Years of early-morning TV appearances have taught me tried-and-true tricks to reduce under-eye luggage. Sounds gross, but a thin layer of Preparation H hemorrhoid cream under the eyes will shrink swelling within five minutes. Witch-hazel-soaked cotton pads also reduce swelling and irritation. Steep bags of green tea in warm water and press on tired eyes. Follow with cold spoons to decrease swelling.

ADVICE FROM THE A-LIST

Tim Quinn
Celebrity makeup artist, Giorgio Armani Beauty

My favorite trick for covering dark circles or discolorations on the face is to use a combination of pink corrector and your personal concealer shade and make tiny vertical "stripes" under the eye, then blend with a concealer brush. I do this after applying eye makeup so that you don't risk any eye shadow or mascara smudges. Start with the pink corrector close to the inner corner of the eye, and alternate stripes.

Six Ways to Boost Radiance at Home

One of the hardest things about pregnancy is relinquishing control. You may not be able to control your body, but you can still exert a smidgeon of type A behavior by managing your skin. A preventative regime can ward off a host of hormone-induced problems.

1. Start with a low-lather, oil-based cleanser. Best Bets: Cetaphil Gentle Daily Cleanser, Kinerase, B. Kamins Vegetable Skin Cleanser, Dr. Hauschka Cleansing Milk, Burt's Bees Orange Essence Facial Cleanser or Soap Bark Chamomile Deep Cleansing Cream, Avalon Organics, Sonya Dakar Red Grapefruit Wash.

2. To pump up the luster factor, exfoliate three times per week. Exfoliation maximizes product penetration, encourages cellular turnover, and can ward off melasma.

3. You may not be knocking them back these days, but customizing a "cocktail" of products (beauty parlance for layering a variety of gentle but active products for increased efficacy) for the face and décolleté is integral to great skin. Also, moisturizing throughout the day (over makeup) keeps skin hydrated and supple.

4. Invest in an antioxidant-rich eye cream and a creamy moisturizer. Again, think about the fetus. You need to supplement moisture-boosting elements to help your skin's ability to stay hydrated. Key ingredients to look for are peptides, caffeine, hyaluronic acid, and omega-3, 6, and 9 fatty acids.

5. Toss on a nourishing mask while chilling out in the tub. Essential-oil extracts and vitamins will boost hydration and plump the skin's surface.

6. Whether you live in Miami or Anchorage, sunblock is key. Sun exposure at any time of the year encourages hyperpigmentation, which is very difficult to eradicate post-delivery. Look for brands with UVA and UVB protection that contain titanium dioxide and zinc.

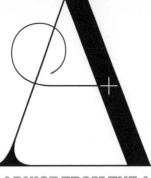

Kate Somerville
Celebrity aesthetician

Think of your skin as a garden. You've got to *weed, seed, feed,* and *water* to get skin glowing again!

1. WEED! Start by getting rid of the junk. Sweep away dead skin cells and clean clogged pores by using an enzyme-based exfoliant. Do this about three times a week.

2. SEED! Use a mineral mask to tighten pores, balance skin, and deliver essential minerals to cells. Look for black silt mud or natural clay masks.

3. FEED! Slather the skin in vitamins and antioxidants to brighten and lighten post-pregnancy pigmentation. Look for vitamins C and E to get the job done.

4. WATER! Pump your skin with hydration. Topically, use products with hyaluronic acid, and internally, bump up moisture levels with omega-3 supplements, such as flaxseeds.

Pregnancy-Specific Products

Feel stressed about questionable ingredients? Pregnancy-specific skin-care products go that extra mile to ensure that they are free from all things toxic. One of my favorites, Mama Mio, has a "No Nasties" policy, meaning that its products are free from synthetic colors, parabens, sulfate detergents, petrochemicals, and a host of known irritants. Developed by a triumverate of British supermamas, Mama Mio puts a playful spin on the woes of maternity with Boob Tube Firming Cream, Tummy Rub Stretch Mark Butter, and Wonder-Full Balm.

Gabby Reece's Crave-Curbing Smoothie

It's tough to get that steak, chicken, and broccoli down during those early stages of pregnancy. The problem? Sugar cravings are born of a lack of protein. Start your morning off with a nutritionally balanced smoothie that tastes great and gives you the stamina to say no to Mr. Butterfinger. Here's what you need: Catie's dissolvable organic greens (as directed), 8 ounces rice or almond milk (vanilla or chocolate), protein powder (CytoSport's Muscle Milk), 1 teaspoon ground flaxseed, 1 cup frozen fruit, 1 banana, ½ teaspoon peanut butter or almond butter. See Gabby's site (www.thehoneyline.com) for more healthful recipes.

BEAT THE BARF No matter how you accessorize, the preggo heaves are tough to chicify. The best you can do is to be prepared. Ginger tea, candied ginger, motion wristbands, acupuncture on the forearm, and constant quaffs of seltzer with lemon help to keep nausea at bay. If you have the misfortune of being what I call Puke-ahontas, be sure to keep small plastic bags, a travel toothbrush and paste, breath mints, and tissues in your purse at all times.

Diet: Feed Your Face

What you eat impacts your complexion. Though it seems obvious, derms emphasize that great skin is contingent upon a nutritious diet and downing eight 8-ounce glasses of water per day. You don't need to axe them from your diet, but know that dehydrating coffee, fried foods, and salt incite toxicity (which dulls skin), zits, and under-eye swelling.

All through college, as I subsisted on a steady diet of popcorn, yogurt, and cinnamon-raisin bagels, I wondered . . . Why, oh why am I permanently constipated? My mom, a reasonably healthy eater, did not divulge the wisdom that is pooping protocol: Starches + veggies + fruit = a satisfying trip to the bathroom. Okay, you're wondering, where is this going? Here's the point: For me, the carb-heavy diet of pregnancy recalled those painful bouts of constipation. And constipation affects the condition of your skin, causing breakouts and blotchiness.

KEEP IT MOVING: THREE TIPS FOR
CONSTIPATION RELIEF

1. A diet rich in fiber, antioxidants (sweet potato, broccoli, spinach, almonds, carrots, berries, whole grains) will boost the immune system, increase cellular turnover, and make you poop.

2. If tropical fruits such as kiwi, mango, papaya, and melon are nature's brooms, spinach and broccoli are its Dustbusters.

3. Sprinkle ground flaxseed into salads and cereal. When ground, this nutty-flavored source of essential fatty acids gives reticent bowel movements a hard-to-resist come-hither.

MAKEUP: FAUX GLOW 101

Like fashion, the beauty component of pregnancy is about accenting the good and camouflaging the unsightly. When I awaken (pregnant or not), I am sallow and baggy-eyed. By the time I caffeinate and walk out the door for work, my skin tone is even and, dare I say it, radiant. Dewiness and a soft, healthy-looking glow are a direct result of neutralizing discolorations and blending foundation with light-reflective particles. So when friends praise my "perfect" skin, I chuckle and award myself high marks for cosmetic craftiness. To achieve the goddess-like perfection of, say, Jennifer Lopez, yank a page from the playbook of celebs' glam squads and become a master of calculated subtlety.

Shimmer Product

Radiant celebrities should all give a hearty thank-you to shimmer powder in their Oscar acceptance speeches. Applying shimmer product (it comes in a creamy blush, powder, or lotion format) to the apple of the cheeks, the nose, the forehead, and the eyelids will give you that insta-luminescence of red-carpet luminaries.
BEST BETS: Dior Poudre Shimmer; Smashbox Softlights; Revlon Skinlights

Bronzer

Bronzer is the eighth wonder of the world. The moment that you feel sallow and unattractive, apply bronzer to your face, décolleté, and other exposed areas. The result: a sun-kissed just-been-to-St. Bart's-glow will lift your mood instantly.
BEST BETS: Lancôme Star Bronzer; Physicians Formula Bronzing Veil; Guerlain Terracotta Light

HOT TIP
Coating on too much foundation, powder, and bronzer will leave you looking like a tragic eighties Cake-and-Bake (see Preggo Glossary) victim.

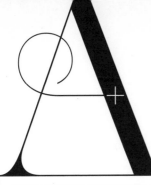

Jean Godfrey-June
Beauty editor, *Lucky*

I don't look like I wear a lot of makeup; neither do most other beauty editors I know. That would be the whole point of makeup, would it not? The idea is you but better: your eyes, but a little bigger, a little more entrancing. Your skin, but with fewer blemishes/wrinkles/blotches. Your lips, but just a tint-y bit more colorful, shiny, and appealing. Anyway, on a typical day (pregnant or no), my no-makeup look involves the following:

• self-tanner
• tinted moisturizer
• under-eye concealer
• mascara
• gel eyeliner
• oil-blotting sheets
• well-groomed eyebrows

If I'm feeling especially in need of a little extra, I use a little cream blush, but this step is rarely taken, for reasons I don't understand. **NOTE:** I am not one for a long-lasting lip product. I enjoy putting it on and on and on, and the color and texture I strive for is "barely there." I always have at least three imperceptibly different tint/balm/gloss/sheer lipstick varieties rattling around in my bag, so as to be able to constantly change my look without changing my look.

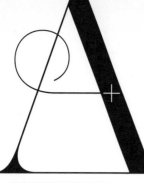

ADVICE FROM THE A-LIST

Tim Quinn
Celebrity makeup artist,
Giorgio Armani Beauty

I always advise applying in the shape of a 3. Starting at the temples, follow along and slightly under the cheekbone to the apples of the cheek, then finish along the jawline—and finally dust in the shape of a cross down the center and across the face—this way there is still a play of light and contour to the face. It looks more natural and not so flat as just swirling bronzer all over.

Face Oil

For increased dewification, work face oil into the palms of your hands and gently pat it into the skin. The oil softens lines and wrinkles and gives a subtle glow. This can be done at any point during the day, even over makeup, when you feel dry.

BEST BETS: Bobbi Brown "Extra" Oil; Decleor Aromessence Iris; Dr. Hauschka Normalizing Oil

Color Corrector

Serious bags need serious camouflage. Whatever your ethnicity, combining color corrector—a pink-, peach-, yellow-, or green-hued cream—with concealer (slightly lighter than your skin tone) can reduce that purple/blue bruised look under the eyes. For more precision, use a concealer brush to blend. I'm a fan of the twofer that packages concealer and color corrector together.

GUIDE TO COLOR CORRECTORS

YELLOW Best to combat red blotchiness, pimples, or broken capillaries around the nose.

GREEN Masks red patches like rosacea.

PEACH AND PEACHY PINK Cover the purplish bruised look resulting from exhaustion and nausea. This works for most complexions and ethnicities.

NOTE: All ethnicities can benefit from color corrector. Pop by a department-store counter for advice about what shade works with your coloring.

BEST BETS: Bobbi Brown Corrector; Armani Master Corrector; Laura Mercier Secret Camouflage

Faux Glow 101:
A Cheat Sheet
Adiós, hormonal skin, hello radiance!

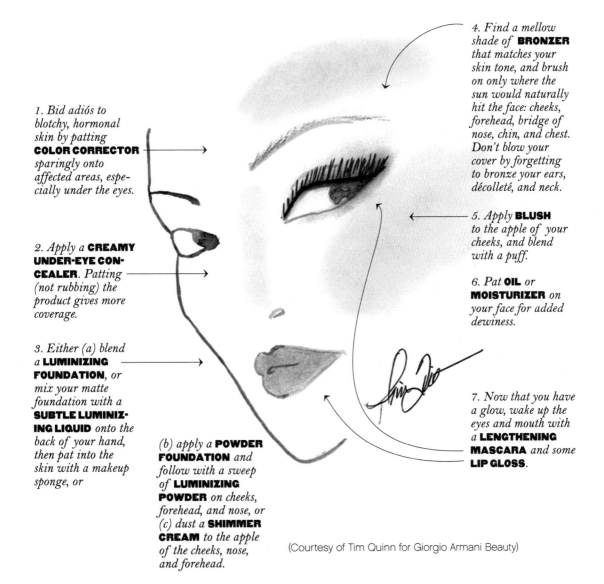

1. Bid adiós to blotchy, hormonal skin by patting **COLOR CORRECTOR** *sparingly onto affected areas, especially under the eyes.*

2. Apply a **CREAMY UNDER-EYE CON-CEALER**. *Patting (not rubbing) the product gives more coverage.*

3. Either (a) blend a **LUMINIZING FOUNDATION,** *or mix your matte foundation with a* **SUBTLE LUMINIZ-ING LIQUID** *onto the back of your hand, then pat into the skin with a makeup sponge, or*

(b) apply a **POWDER FOUNDATION** *and follow with a sweep of* **LUMINIZING POWDER** *on cheeks, forehead, and nose, or (c) dust a* **SHIMMER CREAM** *to the apple of the cheeks, nose, and forehead.*

4. Find a mellow shade of **BRONZER** *that matches your skin tone, and brush on only where the sun would naturally hit the face: cheeks, forehead, bridge of nose, chin, and chest. Don't blow your cover by forgetting to bronze your ears, décolleté, and neck.*

5. Apply **BLUSH** *to the apple of your cheeks, and blend with a puff.*

6. Pat **OIL** *or* **MOISTURIZER** *on your face for added dewiness.*

7. Now that you have a glow, wake up the eyes and mouth with a **LENGTHENING MASCARA** *and some* **LIP GLOSS**.

(Courtesy of Tim Quinn for Giorgio Armani Beauty)

Channel Your Inner Fashion Editor

Nothing frumps you up like . . .
sneakers . . . droopy boobs . . .
orthotic-looking
footwear . . . matchy outfits . . .
too-long hemlines . . . two-toned
hair . . . a lack of glitz . . .
oversized Michelin Man
clothing . . . anything that could
resemble your mother's
pregnancy outfits (unless, of
course, she was Mia Farrow's
doppelgänger) . . .

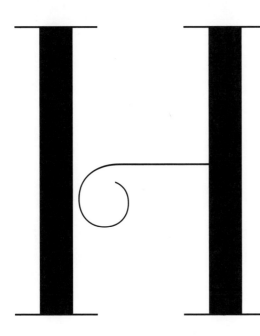urrah!! Le Bump has arrived. You can finally show-case your belly to the world. You have about seven to fifteen extra pounds at this point. Your goal? To avoid the Easy Spirit-meets-jumbo-velour-tracksuit scenario at all costs. Each day, as you heave your ever-expanding frame from bed, challenge yourself to design an outfit so fabulous that no fewer than ten people will comment on how divine you look. **Creating a great outfit, pregnancy or not, is like painting a picture.** You start with a basic, your canvas, and build it up with images, color, and texture. Once you've captured the desired "look," you go back and introduce

the requisite accents to make a complete statement. But any fashion editor worth her Jimmy Choos will tell you that a fresh look requires new perspective, not a new canvas. **By simply rotating basic silhouettes and layering with groovy accessories, you can create dozens of killer looks.** Translation? You don't need thirty different garments for a month's worth of maternity outfits.

ESTABLISH YOUR LOOK: PLAY UP YOUR ASSETS

With your belly busting triumphantly from restraining waist-bands, this is the time to evaluate your body type (see page 111) and establish your personal pregnancy "look."

Do you have big boobs? A thick midsection? A generous rear? Sky-high supermodel gams? Body type figures heavily into whether the cut of a garment, or "silhouette," will be flattering or not. Case in point: Just because you loved the way a crisp white button-down hugged Halle Berry's hourglass bod does not mean that that the white button-down will deliver the same sexy secretary look to you. Spend time determining the shapes that play up your assets and play down your least favorite body parts. These flattering silhouettes—the wrap dress; the jewel-neck slip dress; a deep V-neck top with slimming black maternity trousers; a tunic, jeans, and a flowy knit—will become your "uniform," the foundation of your pregnancy wardrobe.

Have fun with your bodacious newfound curves. Flaunt your belly and boobs in a Lycra dress. Cast nightgowns as ready-to-wear. Yank your favorite maxi skirt over your ample chest and craft a stellar sleeveless dress. Then tap into your inner fashion editor to "bump up" these basics into looks that amplify the bravado of your bump.

Make your swanlike neck the focal point with shoulder-grazing chandelier earrings. Use a high-octane elasticized belt just under your boobs to add color and create the suggestion of a waistline. Make like a celebrity and layer Victorian pendants with a few gold chains on every outfit to add verticality and a dose of glitz. Footwear and bags are the pièces de résistance in Preggoville. Style elements to be sure, they also provide proportion by elongating the silhouette and visually balancing the bump.

HOT TIP
Three universally flattering ways to play up your assets:
• a shorter hemline
• a lower décolletage-baring neckline
• a heel

You don't need dozens of garments. With creativity, confidence, and a cadre of cool accessories, you can transform a handful of items into dozens of jaw-dropping looks. The most important ingredients to preggo chic? Creativity and confidence.

AU REVOIR TOUGH CHIC, HELLO, SOFT SILHOUETTES: HOW TO EMBRACE ETHEREAL LAYERING WITHOUT LOSING YOUR EDGE

If you are a card-carrying member of the Victoria Beckham school of leather and skintight power jackets, you may have to relinquish your austere duds for a softer style, at least for a few months. For the most part, structured, form-fitting clothing—sharply tailored nipped-and-tucked jackets, tight, straight-leg trousers, blazers equipped with power shoulders—are far too restrictive to withstand the massive bloatage of pregnancy. Here's a guide: "Structured," "severe," "architectural," and "hard" refer to garments that deliver a crisp, sexy Dietrichesque silhouette. You, my fine ladies, should revel in garments that are more Stevie Nicks ethereal with soft, billowy fabrication. Think deconstruction, flowy silhouettes without definition of the shoulders and waist. Soft does not mean sloppy. Designers such as Dries Van Noten, Issey Miyake, DKNY's Pure collection, Comme des Garçons, Yohji Yamamoto, and Zero + Maria Cornejo have made nonstructured garments a hallmark of their careers. These clothes skim the body and create a more slouchy/sporty elegance. Of course, you can always add some tough-cookie elements to your look with Wow Factor accessories (see page 66): skull-and-crossbone scarves, biker boots, and a studded bracelet.

CHIC EXPECTATIONS }

One of my favorite designers before, during, and after pregnancy is the Doyenne of Drape, Maria Cornejo. Known for her uneven hems and bubble shapes, she has in-the-know editors flocking to her NYC shop for architectural "before and after" pieces. Here, Cornejo's pregnancy uniform—drapey bubble tunics and a cotton crop knee "beetle" pant—marries high style with functionality. (Courtesy of Maria Cornejo)

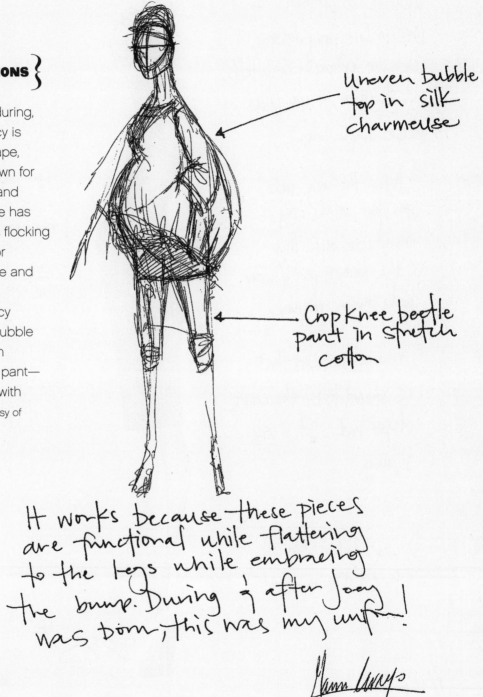

Uneven bubble top in silk charmeuse

Crop knee beetle pant in stretch cotton

It works because these pieces are functional while flattering to the legs while embracing the bump. During & after Joan was born, this was my uniform!

While I was pregnant, I _lived_ in knit jersey dresses, which are extremely comfortable and _stylish_ too, if you follow these simple rules:

1) Define the area under your bust, all the way around your back. This is the narrowest part of your body during pregnancy!

2) Find a dress cut that is shaped to fit the curve of your back. It is _very_ slimming.

3) Wear darker colors, they have a slimming effect!

Milly

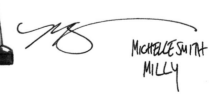

{ **THE LBD** While pregnant, Milly designer Michelle Smith channeled Audrey Hepburn with a uniform of sleek LBDs. This image illustrates the _kapow_ impact of a body-skimming dress that hugs the contour of the back and creates a flattering silhouette through strategic "empire waisting."
(Courtesy of Michelle Smith)

MICHELLE SMITH
MILLY

BACK IN BLACK

There is a reason that, each season, editors declare that "black is the new black." Black is mysterious and chic. Black is basic enough to make a statement. Or not. Black is classic. Black is seasonless. Black matches everything. Black can be dressed up or down. Most important? Because it absorbs light, black hides imperfections and is, hands down, the most slimming color on the planet. For a pregnant woman, black is the ultimate neutral and should be the foundation of the wardrobe (see "The Uniform," p. 57). Pregnant women need the perfect LBD (little black dress). Depending upon how large you are, you may want a maternity-specific LBD; a black skirt, black leggings, black tights (for winter pregnancy), and a super-long black Lycra tank top to layer under everything. Look for "now and later" items. For my two black dresses, I was able to go up a few sizes and buy a simple slip dress and a stretchy number. These pieces still work for me today.

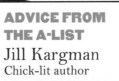

ADVICE FROM THE A-LIST

Jill Kargman
Chick-lit author

ON HER LOVE OF BLACK
My uniform? Black, black, and a bit more black. I liked tighter stuff that showed I was knocked up and not just obese. Instead of maternity clothing, I shopped the fat section of stores like Urban Outfitters and H&M. I lived in all those baby-doll dresses like Marc by Marc Jacobs, but instead of belting them, I let them just go A-line and added leggings or thick black tights and black boots.

BUMP IT UP: THE ABCS OF GARMENT ROTATION

Fashion editors, the women behind the most influential magazine shoots, are mix masters extraordinaire. They can take a basic sheath dress and whip it into a WASP Princess (pearls + slingbacks + classic cardigan), Downtown "It" Girl (cropped vintage leopard jacket + ankle boots + jangle of gold pendants), or Snappy CEO (tweed jacket + diamond studs + pumps) by skillful layering and accessorizing. *Bump It Up* takes the editorial concept of garment rotation and fine-tunes it for pregnancy. The formulaic philosophy—reworking and super-accessorizing versatile basics—diminishes the inherent stress of pregnancy dressing. And it proves that having style results from mixing and matching compelling accent pieces, not piling on expensive brand names.

The system is simple. Women establish the Uniform, four to five easy and flattering silhouettes comprising maternity and non-maternity basics: a bias-cut jersey dress, a black empire-waist dress, the black pencil skirt, jeans, a long black tank top, a navy shirtdress. These basics are groovified with punchy shawls, swingy print jackets, and other eye-catching Add-ons. Dynamic accessories—gold bangles, tribal beads, cocktail rings, exotic belts—are what infuses each look with the Wow Factor.

super-accessorizing

\ ('sü-pər ik-'se-sə-rī-ziŋ) \ *n.* \ fashion term for amping up a basic garment by piling on eye-catching jewelry, handbags, shoes, and scarves.

Here's the formula:

- Craft your anchor outfits to function as the Uniform.
- Enhance the Uniform with dazzling Add-ons.
- Inject your look with Wow Factor by adding fabulous accessories.

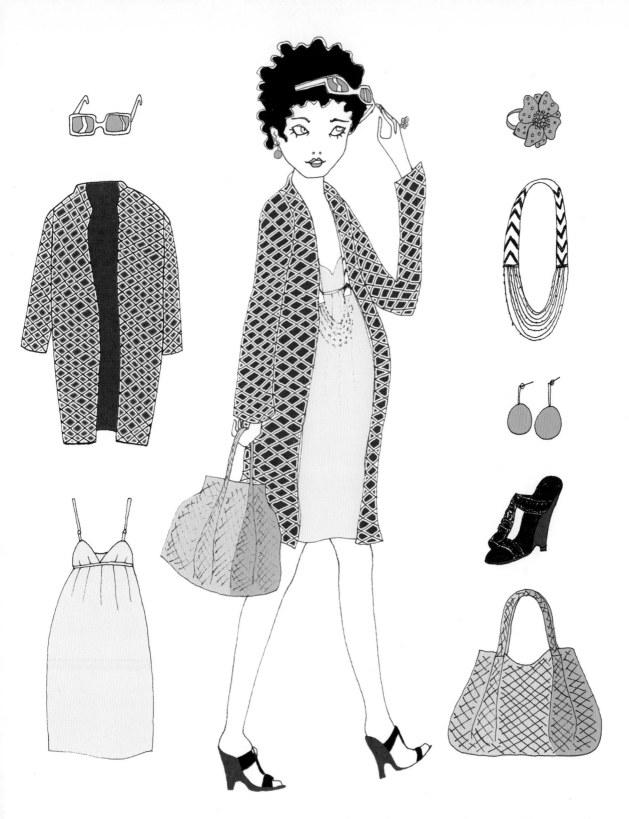

Miracle Garment!
The Wolford Havana Tank Top

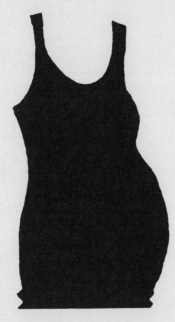

This stretchy, extra-long black Lycra tank top (see page 58) is to pregnancy what mustard is to hot dogs. One cannot exist without the other. Complete codependence. The straps are the perfect width—sexy yet wide enough to accommodate a support bra. The length is long enough to take you through the pregnancy. The cotton-nylon-elastyne blend does not pill. I wore the same Wolford tank three times a week throughout both of my pregnancies.

THE UNIFORM

When Donna Karan debuted her "Seven Easy Pieces" collection in 1985, I was transfixed. Interchangeable basics that work day or night! Donna's revolutionary system of dolling up basics made getting dressed effortless and accessorizing a must. Already a flea-market fiend, I immediately plugged my high school treasure trove—rhinestone baubles, white Ray-Bans, hippie belts, and tatty Salvation Army jackets—into a low-rent version of Donna's concept. It was crystal clear: Accessories create attitude. Similar to DK's concept, the Uniform comprises versatile, seasonless essentials, a combination of nonstructured civilian clothing and must-have maternity items that work for every occasion. These dress-them-up, dress-them-down silhouettes, along with the breezy pieces from trimester 1 (tunics, empire-waist dresses, shifts, and trapeze dresses) are the tabula rasa of your pregnancy wardrobe. Add-ons and Wow Factor are the style elements that coolify basics commensurate with your bump.

ADVICE FROM THE A-LIST
Rae Ann Scandroli Herman
Accessories editor, *Glamour*

An edited wardrobe of functional basics makes it easier to get dressed in the morning. It's like a uniform. I had five silhouettes—a stretchy maternity pencil skirt, Citizens of Humanity maternity jeans, black maternity trousers, Vince V-neck sweater dresses, a black dress. The trick to making minimal basics seem like a closet full of great looks is to mix and match with dramatic accessories like belts, big necklaces, oversized totes, and groovy costume jewelry (cuff bracelets, pendants, cocktail rings). Lighten the mood with colorful scarves and some print. I wore animal-print shoes to break up my neutral palette.

THE UNIFORM MUST-HAVES: ON NEUTRAL GROUND

Neutrals are fashion chameleons that take on the mood of whatever garments they're layered with. Your neutral (mostly black) basics can be mixed and matched to work for anything from a cocktail party to a trip to Wal-Mart.

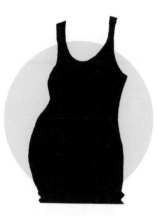

←A super-long black Lycra tank top

This is an essential layering piece for jeans and skirts. The longer bump-enhancing tanks are chic on their own and allow you to wear cropped sweaters and jackets.

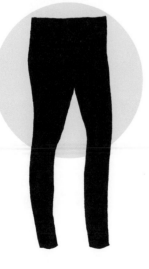

←Black leggings

The perfect slimming foil for a voluminous top or dress.

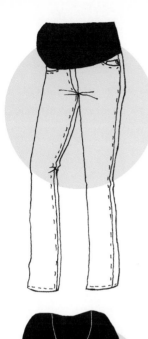

←Dark denim pregnancy jeans

Just as you would in your civilian life, dress them up with heels and boots or slip on ballet flats.

←Soft, jewel-neck, to-the-thigh tees in white and black

Wear them alone or layered under shorter pieces.

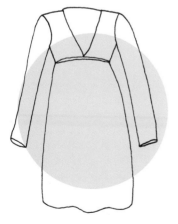

←The empire-waist dress

Strapless or with sleeves, this is still your pal. The shape accentuates the rib cage and disguises bottom heaviness.

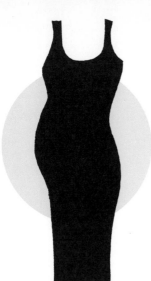

←A basic black jersey bias-cut dress

It flatters most body types and can be worn fifty different ways. Jersey is a dream fabric. It is wrinkle-free, breathable, and has the unique ability to stretch with you.

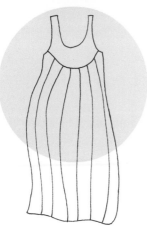

←A maternity black stretchy pencil skirt

This can take you to the office and out to dinner. The waistband can be folded over to turn it into a miniskirt.

←Above-the-knee shifts

Cute, comfy, and au courant. This silhouette enhances the cute pregnant-chick factor in a major way. Vintage slips make great shifts.

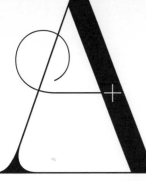

ADVICE FROM THE A-LIST
Filipa Fino, accessories editor, *Vogue*

SEVEN TIPS FOR SAILING THROUGH PREGNANCY WITH PANACHE

1. Super-accessorize basics with fun, dramatic pieces.

2. Invest in thin stretch-cotton basics like tees and dresses.

3. Stock up on Spanx underwear—it holds your belly button in.

4. Have your tailor open up trouser seams at the side and put rubber bands in. You can have them removed later.

5. Think lean: Have six great basics to work with, and punch them up: Underlay and overlay jewelry, belt a sleek cardigan under the bump, carry big bags.

6. Wear empire-waist, A-line, and shift dresses, because they flatter a pregnant body.

7. Don't be afraid of happy colors and prints.

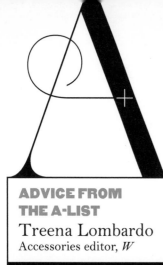

ADD-ONS

This is where we tap into whimsy and trends. Whereas the Uniform is your "blank slate" of staples, Add-ons are all about color, texture, and contrast. Layering your fade-into-the-background basics with statement-making elements serves two functions: electrifying basics with *your* personal style and disguising the fact that you are rotating the same garments day in and day out. What to look for? Pieces that liven up a muted palette. Unstructured knits in electric colors add zing to a basic dress. Bouclé jackets are genteel. A three-quarter-length jacket is at once sporty and cosmopolitan. Upbeat prints—geometric, black and white, or colorful swirls à la Pucci—are eye-catching enough to take the focus from that black Lycra dress that you've worn out for every evening event since January. A marigold trench adds sophistication to trousers or a dress. A slouchy boyfriend jacket over a vintage slip is the epitome of urban glam. Animal print says "racy." And a va-va-voom fur jacket drips Parisian je ne sais quoi. Whatever the season, shawls and wraps (cotton, linen, wool, or cashmere) are both functional and fashionable, introducing pops of color and texture to basics. They can be draped around the shoulders, bunched up around the neck, or wound simply, traipsing elegantly over the shoulder.

ADD-ON MUST-HAVES

So whether you are tall, short, or round, black is the cornerstone of your pregnancy uniform. To make your look pop, tap into eye-catching Add-ons. Layering the following silhouettes provides easy style that is at once sporty and chic.

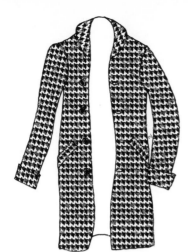

←The three-quarter-length jacket

A favorite of A-list designers, this elegant A-line jacket bumps up basics with Euro fab flair. Wear the to-the-knee jacket (fabricated for every season in silk, linen, boiled wool, and cotton) with a shorter black dress, trousers, or jeans. It looks especially great in a print or bold color.

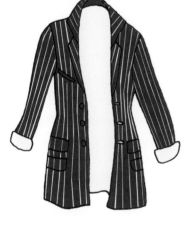

←The boyfriend jacket

Sporty and attractively gender-bending, the subtly structured boyfriend jacket features a slim cut, nipped waist, and lapels. The thigh length makes it a nice counterpoint to a soft, mid-thigh dress.

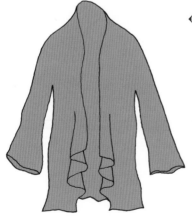

←The unstructured knit

Slouchy, slick, flowy, or fitted, knits offer a soft silhouette that is both chic and cozy for day or evening wear. Get a blast of color with a thin, open-at-the-front cashmere knit sweater or a cable-knit sweater jacket. Wear a silky dress under a roomy wool grandpa sweater. With wide-leg trousers, try a colorful cotton cardigan wrapped and belted over the bump. Knits are crafted for every season and even come in short sleeves to accommodate hot flashes.

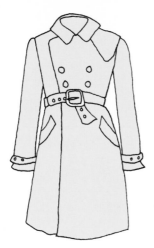

The trench

The classic trench coat, a signature garment of Katharine Hepburn, has been reworked in a rainbow of colors and styles. Belted above the bump or tied in the back, the trench is lightweight and the perfect layering piece. Make sure that it's fitted and hemmed above the knee. A too-long trench will make you look dumpy.

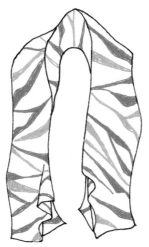

The shawl

Offering both warmth and the perfect pop of color, there is a shawl for every occasion and season. Wear a light linen shawl in lime green with preggo jeans; toss on a pashmina with a black dress; and for the office, drape a vintage floral shawl over a black sweater and pencil skirt.

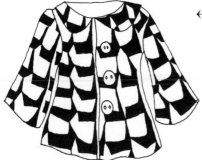

The trapeze jacket

This to-the-hip jacket flares gently out, providing flattering volume. It's a great topper if you're wearing a pencil skirt, leggings, or straight-leg jeans. Add some groove by layering a thin T-shirt that extends farther than the jacket hem.

Miracle Garment!
The Cozy

DKNY hit the *Bump It Up* jackpot with the cozy silhouette. The asymmetrical sweater/shawl is short in the back and long and drapey in the front, making it a versatile (and vertical) layering staple. It can hang open for a fab modern slouchy look with jeans. It can be wrapped and tied or belted over a knee-length dress for a more streamlined look. And because it comes in a variety of colors and fabrications, it translates to every season. The cozy is a perfect example of "now and later" clothing that will take you through the entire nine months of pregnancy and still be a striking classic for years to come.

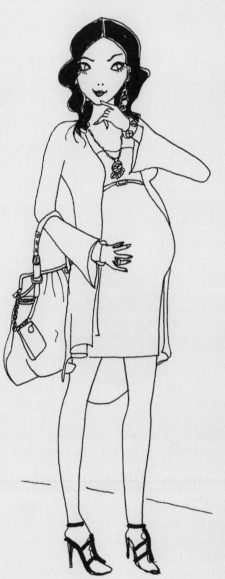

WOW FACTOR

With basics as the foundation of your wardrobe, it's easy to look stale. As my pal Simon Doonan explains, "Dressing down is a crime against humanity." You have layered on some drama, now it's time to master the Wow Factor. Remember, God is in the details. Use accessories (as in WOW!!! Where did she get that insane Egyptian choker????) to amp up your sass. Whether you're conservative or a Gwen Stefani wannabe, work some drama—a boa, lynx, a Lucite cocktail ring, chandelier earrings—into your look. I'm not saying you should walk out of the house dolled up like Cher in Las Vegas. Simply make a statement. Layer on enough flash to bring your basics to life. And when you consider whether or not to buy that metallic handbag, remember that accessories always work. Whether you're thick or thin, accessories are mood amplifiers that add a spring to your step and vitality to your look.

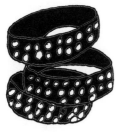

WOW FACTOR MUST-HAVES: DETAIL THERAPY

Bold, beautiful baubles define and refine a look. They also draw your audience's attention away from your cellulite-ridden rump to your incredible eye for detail. Since "Accessories" is a vast and varied category (fashion magazines have editors solely devoted to unearthing the greatest pieces in the industry), I offer you here a rundown of the biggies:

Jewelry

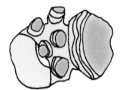

Baubles are the easiest way to make a basic outfit pop. Eclectic accents—think a bunch of Indian bangles, a chain belt, cool Tibetan pendants—add a provocative element to your look. A vintage magnifying glass dangling from a belly-button-length gold chain electrifies that simple black dress and cardigan. A chocolate-brown wrap dress becomes an "It" Girl ensemble with onyx beads, a knuckle duster of a cocktail ring, fishnets over opaque tights, and black boots. Black and white M&M-shaped beads and a fringed lime-green shawl give the black sweater and pencil runway appeal. For a soupçon of *le snob*, don an armful of candy-colored Hermès (or a flea-market knockoff) bangles. News flash: Statement jewelry does not have to cost an arm and a leg. In fact, costume jewelry often gives you the biggest bang for your buck. For trendy pieces at pedestrian price points, stylish women such as Nicole Kidman, Sarah Jessica Parker, and Madonna turn to Kenneth Jay Lane. From wide geometric cuffs and crystal-studded bangles to giant turquoise cocktail rings and jet bead necklaces, Kenneth Jay Lane is one of the fashion industry's top suppliers of oomph.

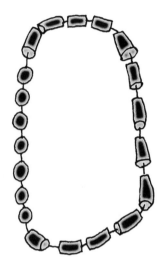

Another way to punch up your look is with vintage accessories (more on this later). Scoop up cuffs, Bakelite necklaces, old-school coin and logo belts at local thrift and vintage stores. My point? Statement jewelry, not delicate charm necklaces or prissy little studs, is what brings an outfit to life.

HOT TIP

If you're having trouble trading in your diminutive gems, try this little experiment. Put on your little black dress with your feminine little choker and wee earrings and take a picture. Then try the same outfit with some oversized beads, giant hoops, and a few black enamel bangles. See what I mean? Store these little pieces of jewelry with your skinny jeans. It will be so much fun to rediscover them after the baby is born.

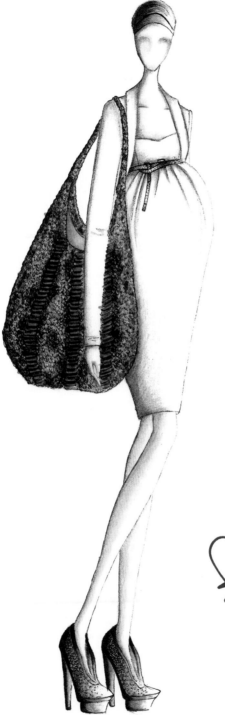

FEMME FERTILE Inspired by super-sophisticated grand dames of fashion, Kroell's sketch embodies the *Bump It Up* ethos, with a turban, an oversized exotic blue bag, sky-high platforms, and a belt snazzily empire-waisting her simple dress and cropped sweater. Her hemline, waist, and huge bag offer pitch-perfect proportion. (Courtesy of Devi Kroell)

Scarves

Silky scarves are another easy way to build up a basic. Forget the old-fart, knotted-under-the-neck country-club look. There is a vast difference between the large rectangular scarves that Granny favors and the attenuated Stevie Nicks/Steven Tyler/Kate Moss–type scarf that drips sensuously down the body. If you take a look at the runway, the thin, extra-long rock-and-roll scarf is all about delivering insta cool. Pair a skull-and-crossbones Alexander McQueen scarf with a T-shirt and jeans. For the office, work a sportif sixties graphic into the look so that it peeks out from inside a slouchy jacket or cardigan. A colorful fringed scarf adds a daring Gypsy Queen element to a black dress.

Bags

A large statement-making tote packs preggo punch. Why? The sheer size balances out your proportion and transports your daily quota of snacks. If you are investing in a quality oversized tote, go for something dark with classic details like eye-catching hardware. For something reflective of seasonal trends, check out "fast fashion" outlets such as Zara, Target, and H&M, where a colorful, of-the-moment handbag can be had for a song.

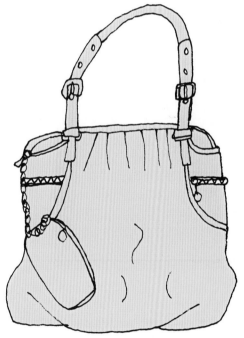

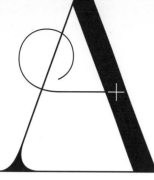

**ADVICE FROM
THE A-LIST**
Aliza Licht
VP of global PR,
Donna Karan International

My major accessories were an elastic DKNY belt and a ribbon belt. I wanted to have a shape during pregnancy, and by belting garments below the boobs, I could transform blah-looking garments into an empire shape. The result? I looked modern, felt thinner, and was far more comfortable than I would have been with a restrictive waistband. I belted my husband's sweaters and his white crisp shirts and paired them with leggings. I belted nonstructured jersey dresses and tunics. It was an easy uniform.

Belts

Pregnancy is the optimal time to discover the joys of belting. If you have a yen for fashion, you'll notice that, on the runway, designers use belts to express the "directionality," or mood, of their collection. Skinny belts feel demure. Chain belts feel sporty. Thicker belts reflect a harder edge. A macramé or leather tie belt screams boho. Aside from being decorative, belts are a functional style element that can make or break a look. A flashy belt below the belly is a way to draw attention to your sumptuous bump and away from other areas that you may not be so fond of at the moment. A stretchy belt can be used below the bra line to create an empire waist. And a thin leather belt can go over a cardigan to add polish.

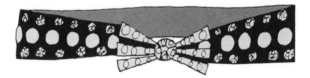

Shoes

A heel visually lengthens your silhouette and, in turn, balances out your tummy-enhanced proportion. Loafers, lace-ups, or any rubber-soled shoes that could double as your octogenarian grandmother's orthotics are verboten. And sneakers are in the same category as sweatpants. Absolutely never, ever, wear sneakers unless you are headed to the gym. You don't need five-inch Carrie Bradshaw stilettos. But with the watermelon in your belly, height will balance out the bulge, elongate your body, and add that soupçon of glamour that transforms dumpy into diva. You will have the most stability with mid-range stacked heels, wedges, and kitten heels. Even cowboy boots offer a great look and excellent support.

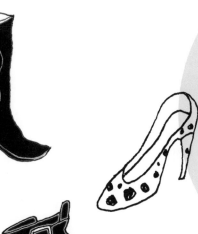

HOT TIP

A pointed toe lengthens the silhouette; a rounded toe gives a stumpier appearance. A form-fitting to-the-knee black boot is essential for a fall/winter pregnancy. The height is a classic, chic style that slims the leg. Summer is the only time that flats are permissible. Flip-flops or cute Grecian sandals are the perfect counterpoint to swingy sundresses.

A SHOE-IN With the cork-soled wedge sandal and chunky, to-the-knee boot, accessories maestro Rafe Totengco gives chic and comfortable footwear options for pregnancy. Note the elongating effect of the woman in boots. Her above-the-knee red coatdress paired with slimming black tights and an oversized tote is modern, comfortable, and totally chic. (Courtesy of Rafe Totengco)

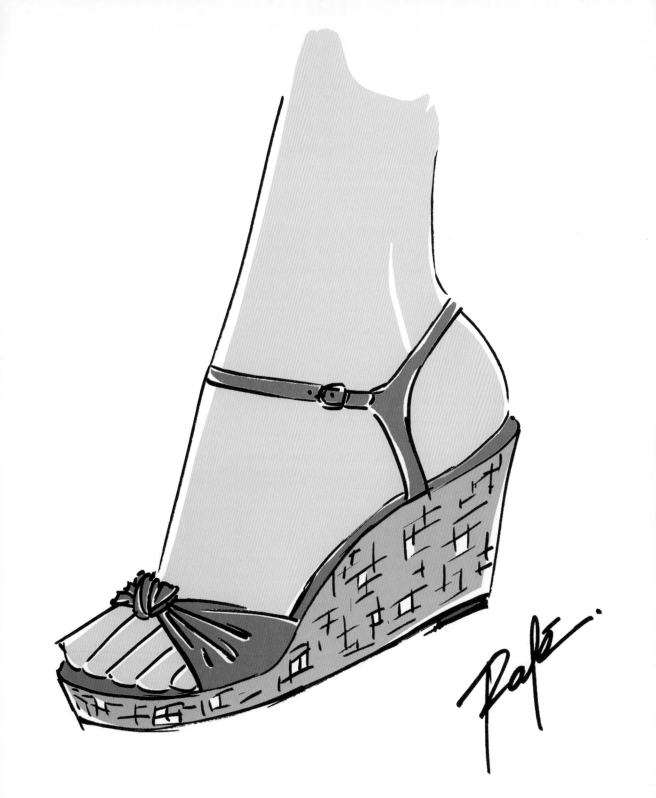

BEWARE THE PEAR: A NOTE ON VOLUME CONTROL

Nothing frumpifies more than oversized clothing and lack of proportion. With the arrival of your bodacious bump, volume control is the key to a balanced, chic look. Some guidelines: If it's big on top, it should be narrow on the bottom. If it's narrow on top, you can add some volume with a skirt or wide-leg pant. Skirts and dresses should be above the knee or sweeping the ground to elongate the body. Legs are slimmed and lengthened with black tights and boots or heels. Big blouses are countered with fitted skirts or tapered trousers. Tailoring is critical.

ADVICE FROM THE A-LIST
Jen Rade
Celebrity stylist to Angelina Jolie, Lisa Rinna, and Pink

ON PROPORTION

Everything you wear during pregnancy should make as much of a statement as your regular wardrobe. You don't need a ton of things; just have great basics and interesting high/low accessories to mix in. Think about proportion once you start showing. Balance a wider bottom with a tight sweater; wear a great legging under a floaty top or tunic. A cool boyfriend blazer (see p. 63) with sleeves rolled up over a tunic and leggings is a super-cute look. Keep lines vertical. Dark colors are more slimming. V-necks lengthen the torso by showing décolletage.

Best bets are amazing leggings (by Fogal or Wolford) that go under the belly, an LBD by Ella Moss or Isabella Oliver, Rachel Pally's soft cotton jersey dresses, T-shirt dresses from American Apparel, "wife-beater" tanks to layer under everything, a great pair of maternity jeans, a trapeze dress, loose-weave, open-front cardigans, a long, fold-down-waistband skirt from James Perse, gauzy, vintage Mrs. Roper caftans, empire-waist dresses.

Every pregnant woman should rent the film *Rosemary's Baby*. Mia Farrow was the most stylish pregnant person. Her look—pixie haircut, ballet flats, leggings, eyelet tunics—created a huge impact on fashion: her proportion was perfect.

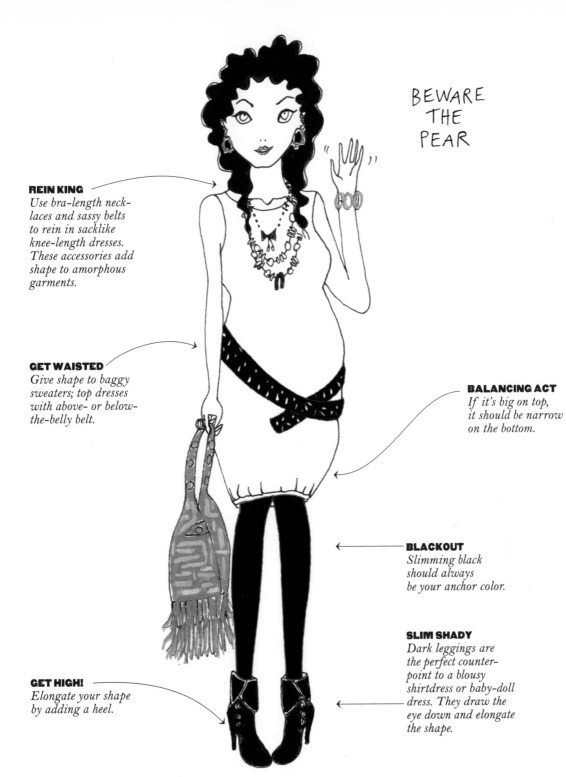

BEWARE THE PEAR

REIN KING
Use bra-length necklaces and sassy belts to rein in sacklike knee-length dresses. These accessories add shape to amorphous garments.

GET WAISTED
Give shape to baggy sweaters; top dresses with above- or below-the-belly belt.

BALANCING ACT
If it's big on top, it should be narrow on the bottom.

BLACKOUT
Slimming black should always be your anchor color.

SLIM SHADY
Dark leggings are the perfect counterpoint to a blousy shirtdress or baby-doll dress. They draw the eye down and elongate the shape.

GET HIGH!
Elongate your shape by adding a heel.

THE ELEVENTH COMMANDMENT: KNOW THY LUXURY PRODUCTS

While hunting down your accent pieces, be aware that adding a fresh twist to a basic wardrobe does not require spending big bucks. Recognize the difference between trendy accent and investment piece. Investment pieces (think a Hermès Birkin, a Loro Piana cashmere cloak, a Van Cleef & Arpels cuff, a Chanel anything) have sustained fashion relevance. They are high-quality "keepers" that will add cachet to your wardrobe for years to come. Trendy accents (think mod vests, super-glitzy tote bags, pink shoes) are whimsical fashion items with a short shelf life (because they are replaced with the next "it" trend the following season). Luckily, we are living in an age of fast fashion, where runway trends are interpreted by inexpensive retailers such as H&M, Zara, and Topshop almost as soon as the last model jumps off the catwalk. Offering directional pieces at bargain-basement prices, these shops are manna for pregnant fashion gals who are committed to injecting of-the-moment elements into their look. A fun printed forty-dollar maxidress a size or two larger, a groovy fifty-dollar faux-fur-trimmed vest, a twenty-dollar neon scarf, and a basketful of glitzy gold jewelry (at $2.99 a pop) will give you major look for a minor investment. And when you regain your slim shape (or simply get sick of these items) you will not be riddled with anger for wasting your hard-earned cash on fashion with a six-month shelf life. The trick is to know thy luxury products and invest with confidence if your purchase is a keeper.

INVESTMENT PIECE   *versus*   TRENDY ACCENT

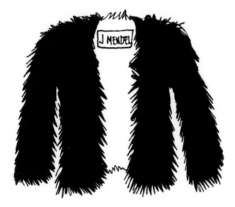

J Mendel fur jacket   vs   faux fur vest from Zara

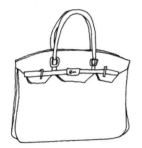

Hermès Birkin bag   vs   neon clutch bag from Topshop

Chanel earrings   vs   glitzy gold jewelry from H&M

TRIMESTER 2 POP QUIZ: TO LEVEL OR NOT TO LEVEL YOUR WALLET

Before you drop a lot of cash on a garment or accessory, ask yourself whether it meets the following five criteria:

1. Am I in love? Am I weak in the knees and will pass out if I don't own this trinket?

2. Is it classic? Is it very high-quality and can be passed down to my daughter or niece?

3. Can I prove that I am not in desperation mode? Do I promise that I will not be sick of this item by spring 2011?

4. Is a knockoff version of this item available at Urban Outfitters, H&M, or Bebe?

5. Am I willing to blow my budget and subsist on Hamburger Helper for the next month?

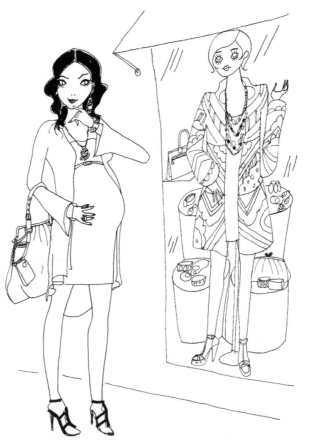

Don't do it!
Desperation Clothing

It happens to all of us. That feeling in the pit of your stomach when you are tragically sick of every item in your closet. Estrogen bubbles in your veins. It can't be put off. You need something new *now*. You descend like a madwoman on your local department store, stalking the aisles for something—anything—to save you from another day in the black shift dress. You spy some pieces with forgiving silhouettes. A flowered peasant blouse! A burnt-orange tunic with Apache beading! Though these pieces would make you retch in a non-preggo state of mind (your finely honed "minimalist architect" look has put the kibosh on color since the early nineties), you toss down your credit card. Back home, these hippie-dippy garments look as out of place as guacamole in India. You wear them a few times and ultimately give them away.

THE TRANSFORMERS

Black is slimming, yes. But too much can be funereal. There are three style elements guaranteed to bump up preggo basics into a look to be reckoned with: a blast of print, a burst of color, and a rendevous with a fabulous piece of fur (real or faux, *bien sûr!*).

1. Color War

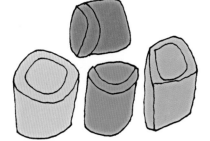

Lift the mood with upbeat pops of color. To many urban warriors, the proposition of comingling "wardrobe" and "color" is unseemly, a nauseating collision of June Cleaver saccharine with Stepford Wife WASP. Let me clarify: The idea is not to dress in color head to toe but rather to use color as an accent, a counterpoint, to your neutral-heavy wardrobe. But there are rules. Just because you like yellow does not mean that you can wear it. This is a mistake many people make and end up looking like a tour guide at Parrot Jungle. The only way to learn what color flatters your complexion is to try things on. If the color warms and enhances your complexion, it works. Conversely, if the image reflected in the mirror bears a strong resemblance to Morticia Adams, 'tis not the hue for you. Once you determine your complimentary colors, pair them with dark basics to energize your look. Wear your multitasking black dress with a red trench. Opt for a brightly colored metallic clutch bag. Try a pumpkin tunic with your black leggings. A colorful scarf adds some style wattage to black trousers and a basic top. Follow in the footsteps of Kate Spade and add small shots of color with a floral brooch, a handbag, shoes, or tights. Jesse Garza, founder of fashion consultancy firm Visual Therapy, feels that pregnancy and bold, daring dashes of neon should go hand in hand. "You have the boobs

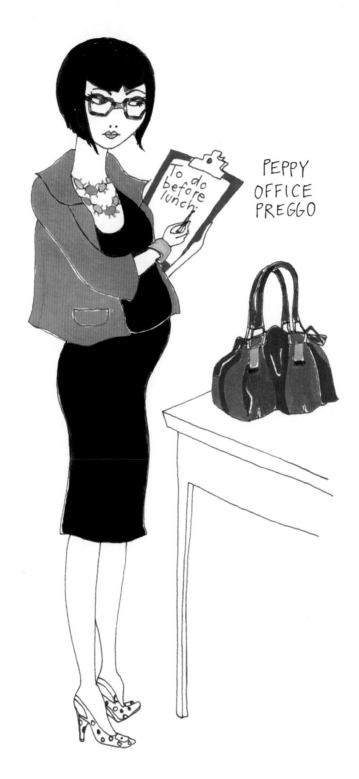

PEPPY OFFICE PREGGO

and the glow going. Why not go avant-garde? Neon is a sexy approach to enhancing a dark color with energy," he explains. "You will definitely stand out in the crowd."

2. Prints Charming

Again, black is a maternity essential, but printed patterns are a fun foil. Wearing prints is very much about finding the patterns that reflect who you are. From kooky graffiti to super-wearable graphics, the options are endless. Mine the animal kingdom. Go Kate Spade/Edie Sedgwick cool with a leopard jacket belted above the bump. Add a racy zebra pump to a black dress. Pair a snakeskin purse and heels with leggings and a long boyfriend jacket (see p. 63). Prints were a major trend in the sixties and seventies. Shop Granny's closet, vintage shops, and flea markets for stylish three-quarter-length jackets (see p. 63), tunics, scarves, and accessories. Replace basic black dresses with an empire-waist maxidress bursting with blossoms. Or a gauzy patterned tunic. *J'adore* all things Caribbean. On a hot summer day, only a breezy caftan (upscale lingerie brands often include delightful gauzy tunics and caftans in their collections) with a sultry jungle print will cool you down. For those who veer modernist, no-nonsense black-and-white prints are always in style. Go artsy with a playful Basquiat-type graffiti print. For a spring and summer pregnancy, it's all about riots of color. And there is the boho fan club, the Nicole Richie type who cannot get enough paisley swirls, ombré, and color blocking. Some designers who excel at prints are Tibi, Diane von Furstenberg, Calypso, Rachel Pally, Missoni, Pucci, Milly, T-Bags, and Nicole Miller.

prints are Great - because they are happy and also they break up the wide area

tunics + leggings were my uniform —

{ STYLEPHILE During her pregnancy, Nicole Miller lived in a uniform of upbeat print tunics with leggings and wedge heels—the perfect marriage of comfort and style. The look is fun and functional because prints add energy and color, breaking up the monotony of an all-black wardrobe. Wedges offer the perfect alternative to spike heels, providing height and comfort. (Courtesy of Nicole Miller)

leggings are so comfortable!

never out of heels → wedges are a good alternative

Nicole Miller

DOWNTOWN
"IT" Girl

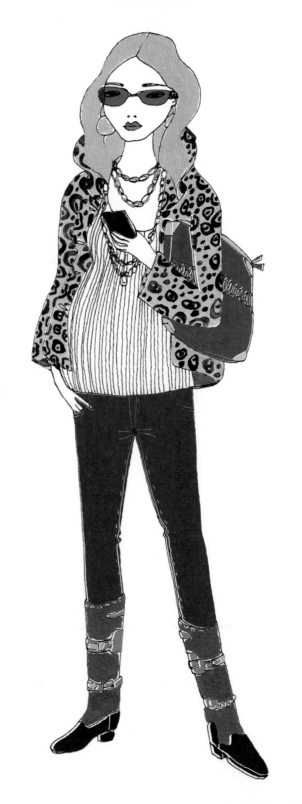

3. Furocious!

Sorry, PETA. Pelts are the ultimate Add-on. Once considered the essence of luxury and old-world aristo chic, fur was worn by glamour gals such as Penelope Tree, Jean Shrimpton, and Edie Sedgwick, paired with thigh-high minis and platforms. For pregnancy, fur (real or faux) puts a luxe spin on basics. Put on your Kate Moss thinking cap and daringly blend this high-end material with low-rent basics. Wear a retro leopard jacket with your preggo jeans and heels. Slip a fabulous fox shawl over a plain black dress. Work a slouchy white rabbit-fur tuxedo jacket over trousers and your Lycra black tank. Again, vintage shops and Granny's closet are great resources.

Homework:
Glamour a-Go-Go

Get your hands on some stacked costumy bangles, a dangly, groovily printed silk scarf, big beads, over-sized sunglasses, some long, gold necklaces, and, say, a gigantic tote bag in orange. Lay your basics out on the bed, place these fetching accessories on top, and watch your outfit pop. That's right. Simple + cool, eye-catching accessories = a polished, statement-making glamorous look.

LET'S GO TO JERSEY!

Once in a while, the fashion world gives us a gift, a fabric that feels as fantastic as it looks. Known for its breathability and ability to stretch with its wearer, jersey tops the preggo popularity charts because it is incredibly comfortable. And flattering. Somehow, jersey drapes perfectly over pregnancy bulges, spotlighting the good and obscuring the nasty. Whether you work in an office, a classroom, or a board-room, this wrinkle-free fabric is a best-bet basic. Jersey comes in a variety of weights and blends, so it is available year-round.

BRAS AND UDDER SUPPORTING ROLES

As your body explodes to Pamela Anderson stature, you need to rein in the twins and remind your belly and butt who's boss.

Bras and Camis

Believe it or not, most women go through pregnancy with the wrong size bra. As a general rule, your bra goes up two cup sizes from pre-pregnancy to nursing. Fit and comfort are essential. First trimester, your breasts are sore but don't change much. By week 16, it's time to get measured by a fit expert (they can be found at most large department stores. One can also have an online fitting session at www.medela.com, maidenform.com, or destinationmaternity.com). Your boobs and rib cage have expanded, so your old bra will not offer enough support. Anne Dimond, majordomo of Bella Materna, the go-to resource for luxury maternity and nursing lingerie, is one such expert. Dimond sums up the need for increased support succinctly: "During pregnancy, your breasts are like a third world bridge. Do you want iffy rope or the security of steel?" If you opt for the latter, she explains, you should wear underwire (with a cup seam behind the breast tissue) and "align your headlights" by physically placing your breasts entirely into the cups. Bella Materna isn't cheap. But the non-pilling, non-fading nylon and Lycra-infused bras do double duty as nursing gear, eliminating the need for a second, "fourth trimester" bra. (In fact, many companies offer multitasking options that take you from trimester 2 through nursing.) And they are available in tough-to-find plus sizes like a G/H cup.

When your civilian cups runneth over, you can also turn to Spanx for support. Spanx's Brallelujah! underwire contour bra is fashioned from sleekifying hosiery fabric, which, aside from being comfortable, eliminates unsightly back fat. The adjustable shoulder and back straps stretch with you, elevating your bountiful bosom from mid-pregnancy through nursing. If your large breasts have turned into "full cup," you will not be relegated to thick World War II nurse–style innerwear. Lilyette and Bella Materna offer sexy, supportive, full-figure bras in traditional, plunge, and strapless styles. Ultra support can also be found in Medela's seamless microfiber bra and Wacoal's Bodysuede underwire bra, which are outfitted with internal "slings" for enhanced lift. If underwire is not your thing, test-drive a smoothing maternity/nursing camisole. Constructed with molded support cups, the camis (which come for small- and large-chested women) are extra long, and rigged specifically for easy-access breast-feeding. For extra support, larger-chested women often layer a tight-fitting camisole over a bra. Representing flat-chested women of America, I was a huge fan of the soft, sports-bra-like "bralets."

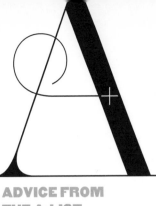

ADVICE FROM THE A-LIST
Liz Smith
National fit expert, Wacoal

One bra won't last forever. You will need a minimum of three bras. This will save you money in the long run and allow your bras to rest. Think one in the wash, one on your body, and one in your lingerie drawer waiting for you. You must rotate your bras to get the most out of them. If you wear the same bra every day, the elastic does not have the chance to recover. Allow approximately one hundred washings and one hundred wearings before your bra needs to be retired.

Brands such as Maidenform, DKNY, Spanx, Hanro, Natori, and Sassybax create sleek underwire-free innerwear that gives support without compression. There is a theory that perky postpartum breasts can be had by defying gravity throughout pregnancy. Yes, that means sleeping in your bra. Yours truly did not sleep in a bra and has retained quasi perkiness. But support 24/7 does make sense. Should you wish to go that route, many of the brands noted above are comfortable enough to be worn to bed.

HOT TIP
Instead of buying a new bra for that last spurt of weight gain and rib-cage expansion, get a hook-and-eye bra extender for your existing bra. It can be removed as you start to lose the baby weight. And yes, the rib cage does go back to the pre-pregnancy setting.

Tights

For a fall/winter pregnancy, dark tights are a great way to elongate the silhouette. Aside from making a fashion statement, maternity specific-tights and pantyhose have a comfy "overbelly" that stretches over your bump and offers increased leg compression to alleviate painful swelling and varicose veins. Assets, the lower-priced brand by the creator of Spanx, offers Marvelous Mama tights and pantyhose designed to "lift one's assets" with slick yarns that slim while providing under-belly and back support. Other quality pregnancy-specific brands are Belly Basics, Gabriella, and Fertile Mind. Many of these brands also have "fashion" leg wear such as fishnets and textured tights for special occasions.

Additional Support

Many women need additional support. The Babybellyband (www.babybellyband.com), Loving Comfort Maternity Support, and Prenatal Cradle (www.prenatalcradle.com) are support systems made of stretchy bands to relieve back and ligament pain associated with pregnancy. The abdominal band is a hard-core girdle that stretches and hooks under the belly. A shoulder-to-groin support harness can be Velcroed on and crisscrossed behind the back to pull the shoulders back and redistribute weight. The groin support helps with prolapsed bladder, painful edema, hernias, and "vulvar varicosities," the dreaded swelling of the vulva. There is also a plethora of maternity belts and bands that reduce pressure in the lower back and offer a smooth look under clothing.

Miracle Product!
Spanx Power Mama Mid-thigh Shaper

This pregnancy-specific shaper (with a cut-out belly for zero compression) allows you to exert that last ounce of control over your growing body. Layered under pants, capris, dresses, and skirts, the shaper hides cellulite, prevents thighs from rubbing together, eliminates VPL (see Preggo Glossary), and provides support to belly and lower back. Assets, Spanx's lower-priced line, offers a less expensive version of the pregnancy-specific shaper called Marvelous Mama Unbelievable Underwear. See www.spanx.com and www.loveassets.com.
(Courtesy of Spanx)

LYCRA, SWEET LYCRA

Now that you have an impressive belly, those clingy fabrics eschewed in the first trimester are cordially invited back to the wardrobe to serve as part of your Uniform. Lycra, the lowbrow material associated with tacky eighties club gear, wins the versatility contest among pregnantistas. Why? Lycra's unique fabrication compresses flab and delivers shape. If it's a quality garment, this sucks-to-the-rib-cage fabric will survive the entire pregnancy by stretching with you. Pound by glorious pound.

HOT TIP
Assets, Spanx's lower-priced line, offers a less costly version of this pregnancy-specific shapewear called Marvelous Mama Unbelievable Underwear. See www.spanx.com and www.loveassets.com.

Contain yourself

with these Lycra essentials:

An extra-long, bump-hugging black Lycra **TANK** (see page 58): This is the ideal topper for almost any skirt or pant. Fashion chameleons, these fade-into-the-background tanks are so plain that, if you pair them with a multitude of punchy partners (see "Add-ons"), nobody will notice that you're wearing the same thing for five out of the seven days in your rotation.

Luxe Lycra **LEGGINGS** (see page 58): An abomination on most women, leggings (not shabby workout gear) are delightfully chic on preggos, a slimming foil to a bump-heavy top. Wear them with blousy tops, tunics, swingy trapeze dresses, and to-the-knee jackets or below-the-bump belted sweaters.

A black mid-thigh Lycra **SKIRT**: This piece can be worn a variety of ways. With the elasticized top folded over just under the belly, you have a sexy mini to wear with a blousy top. The skirt can be worn mid-thigh with the black Lycra top and a printed jacket. Or it can be pulled over the boobs as a tube top.

A bump-hugging black **STRETCHY DRESS**: Fashion brands and retailers from Balenciaga to Target offer takes on this most functional just-above-the-knee dress.

TANKS A LOT
*Soft stretchy tank
tops are a must.*

HIDE AND SLEEK
*A fun scarf can
look chic and
hide the bump!*

THE LOWDOWN
*A low-rise loose-
leg pant can work
for your pregnancy.
They are great
with a tank top or
even with a little
dress over them.*

**{ VA-VA-VOOM
{ VERTICALITY**

Alice + Olivia designer
Stacey Bendet's Uniform?
Stretchy Lycra tops paired
with low-rise, wide-leg
trousers (which she
designed to encompass
her bump). This look is
all about proportion and
verticality. The fitted top
is perfectly balanced by
the gently pleated pant,
which draws the eye down.
The scarf, too, brings
the eye down while slyly
masking the bump.
A heel elongates the look.
(Courtesy of Stacey Bendet)

a l i c e + o l i v i a
Stacey Bendet

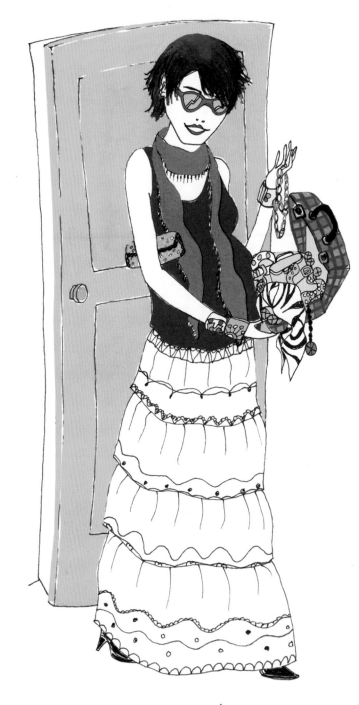

RAID GRANNY'S
CLOSET

VIVA LA VINTAGE

This brings us to my favorite topic: vintage clothing. My favorite homes are designed with a clever combination of antiques and modern pieces, and the same holds true for fashion. For ardent lovers of drama and kitsch, vintage emporiums are the ultimate destination. The one-off vintage pieces—a hot pink Courrèges shift dress, a sugar-spun Galanos chiffon frock, a June Cleaver–type lizard handbag—are the Adds-ons and Wow Factor that will help you and your belly basics stand out in a skinny-jean-and-platform-heel-wearing crowd. And now that the green movement is in full swing, it should be noted that vintage clothing and accessories are environmentally friendly in that they are, more or less, recycled garments.

Scoop up sequined tunics, fringed cashmere wraps, a retro logo belt, and glitzy *Knots Landing*–style jewelry to add pizzazz to pregnancy jeans or black leggings. A silver Lurex knit scarf (Studio 54, anyone?) spices up basic black. The simple, stretchy black V-neck dress (a preggo must-have) is glamified with the addition of a wide fifties coin-studded leather belt and a well-draped, hand-knotted shawl. Your empire-waist dress becomes regal with fabulous chain necklaces, to-the-neck earrings, and Wonder Woman cuffs. Channel Stevie Nicks by introducing a Moroccan Thea Porter jacket to your jeans and Hanes tank. The printed wrap dress is taken to exotic heights with layered agate pendants and a knuckle-duster ring. Comfy caftans, often deemed the essence of dump, get the thumbs-up in a vintage incarnation. Seventies Halston caftans in steaming-hot red are somehow racy. Those bearing ethnic prints are the essence of Upscale Gypsy. Those swirly Pucci-like patterns are the very inspiration for contemporary collections such as BCBG Max Azria. Don't be afraid to merge high and low fashion, like a sequined tunic with Dr. Scholls and jeans. This groovy, eclectic blend is what made Kate Moss a fashion icon. In fact, Kate was my inspiration when I scored a white vintage Ungaro tuxedo jacket for my baby shower. I wore it with a (not so) little black dress and to-the-knee boots. The best part? I still wear that jacket (after tailoring) with my current collections of LBDs (see Preggo Glossary), and it oozes classic cool.

Where, you ask, will I score such glitzy gear? The starting point is always paying a visit to Grandmama (weekend tote in hand) and raiding her closet for old-school goodies. As you tell her what an iconic matriarch she has been to your family, scoop as many eye-catching accents—brooches, belts, necklaces, reptilian bags, and shawls—into your tote as possible. I'm sure that she'll be delighted to contribute to the birth of her grandchild's sense of style. If you can't get to Granny (or the wackadoodle Auntie Mame in your family), swap meets, tag sales, flea markets, thrift stores, and vintage emporiums can be manna for the mama-to-be.

HOT TIP

The most collectible vintage designers are Courrèges, Ossie Clark, Thea Porter, Gucci, Halston, Pucci, Dior, Biba, and Stephen Burrows because their silhouettes and cool fabrications have enduring appeal. These pieces were relatively inexpensive back in the day, so, if you're lucky, Granny may have one socked away in the back of her closet.

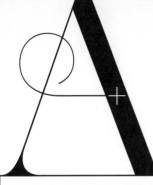

ADVICE FROM THE A-LIST
Cameron Silver
Owner of Decades, Los Angeles's premier vintage boutique

ON HOW TO LOOK SWELL IN VINTAGE

As the belly swells, look for breezy Ossie Clark and Thea Porter pieces. Favored by rock-star wives and other glamour gals, these British designers specialized in dramatic empire-waist silhouettes crafted with groovy fabrics and ethnic prints. For more casual fare, Biba's designs from the seventies are wonderful. The body-skimming dresses and tunics in geometric and art nouveau prints are lightweight, chic, and floaty. Pucci stretch silk jersey dresses—to the knee and floor-grazing—are glam and insanely comfortable. Wrap dresses are easy to find at every price point as they were made by many designers in the seventies. For parties, look for Stephen Burrows, who is known for sexy draped jersey dresses in vibrant colors. Sixties party coats in lamé and prints add glamour to simple black frocks. Breezy V-neck Halston caftans (popularized by Barbra Streisand and Elizabeth Taylor) in layered chiffon or tie-dyed jersey are perfect for lounging about in the final trimester.

VINTAGE ACCESSORIES

Nothing makes a statement quite like an unidentifiable (as in "OMG! That brooch is amazing! Is it early Saint Laurent?") retro accent. Accessories are an easy, inexpensive entry point to vintage. They supply that glam little touch that elevates mere clothing to a look. A quirky woven leather-and-gold belt gives shape to drapey silhouettes. A huge tribal medallion adds panache to a dark caftan. Chain belts deliver polish to a shirtdress and can be adjusted by changing the link closure. Sleek old-school logo belts—think Dior and Gucci from the seventies—are a whimsical under-the-bump flourish. Forget dainty pendants and prissy stud earrings. Jewelry should mirror the bravado of your bump. Bold baubles—cuff bracelets, gold chains, chandelier earrings—amplify your style quotient. Ethnic touches like, say, Masai micro-beaded bracelets, Indian bangles, wooden cuffs, and massive beaded necklaces are unadulterated global glitz. Contrast is achieved by adding pops of print and color with scarves and shawls. Sport them around the neck or trailing artfully over one shoulder. Scarves also make interesting obi belts (over pregnancy-jean panel) or sexy back-baring halter top. And fur, faux or the real deal, is a most chicifying accent. A swingy Kate Moss–ifying leopard jacket for evening is pure Hollywood. (See page 186 for a list of my favorite vintage resources.)

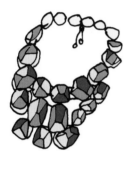

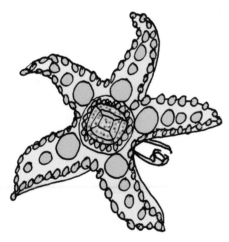

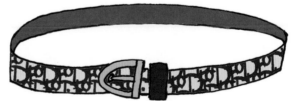

SIGNATURE STYLE 101: HATS OFF TO THE GRAND ECCENTRICS

In high school, while other kids were at band practice, I was at the flea market investing my allowance in rhinestone brooches and fifties bomber jackets. I was into fashion (think Babe Paley meets Madonna) at an early age. But many women don't necessarily have a pre-pregnancy "signature look" to reference. If you have lived for years mystified by runway trends, pregnancy is a golden opportunity to exit your comfort zone and bring your inner glamazon to life. Give a nod to the fashion icons of the twentieth century and use your belly as a VIP pass to the order of eternal divahood. Learn about silhouettes. Discover accessories. Investigate why muses *perenniale*—marvelous **Marchesa Luisa Casati**, dynamic **Diana Ross**, chic social-ite **Babe Paley**, sixties siren **Edie Sedgwick**, boho babe **Talitha Getty**, and art deco diva **Nancy Cunard**—became style revolutionaries. These histrionic women (who, by the way, would rather have swept donkey dung than be deemed average in any way) created a unique brand of outré glamour. They were gaga for art and lived life unfettered by convention. Their devil-may-care lifestyle was evidenced in idiosyncratic fashion choices: gowns as day wear, turbans, shoulder-sweeping earrings, extreme eye makeup, stacked-to-the-elbows bangles, cloaks fashioned of peacock feathers. I am not suggesting that you go radical. Your task is to find a scintillating look that suits your personality and flatters your body type. Upper East Side Lady Who Lunches? Downtown "It" Girl? Haute Hippie? Groovy Gal About Town? Be the girl with the Bakelite cuff bracelets and fabulous YSL scarves adorning every outfit. Wear

Grandma's Lurex sweater sets to the supermarket. Layer vintage Betsey Johnson baby-doll dresses with Byzantine beads and rhinestone crosses just because. The larger you feel, the more accessories required. Your Cinderella moment awaits!

Homework:
Amp Up Your Fashion Cognition

Take a tutorial (from the comfort of your couch) in high style by observing the social swans, groovy gamines, and daredevil divas in these "fashion moment" TV shows and films: Rosalind Russell and Joan Crawford in *The Women*, Mia Farrow in *Rosemary's Baby* and *The Great Gatsby*, Audrey Hepburn in *Funny Face* and *Breakfast at Tiffany's*, Catherine Deneuve in *Belle de Jour*, Marlene Dietrich in *Shanghai Express*, Meryl Streep in *The Devil Wears Prada*, and Joan Collins in *Dynasty*.

RETHINK YOUR WARDROBE: SKIRTS AS DRESSES, DRESSES AS TUNICS, AND INNER WEAR AS OUTERWEAR

Just because something does not fit the way it was intended doesn't mean it must be banished from Bumpland. Creativity is the lifeblood of fashion. Rethinking your wardrobe takes the concept of multitasking clothing to the next level. Which will, in turn, save you cash.

Skirts as Dresses

My bodacious preggo bod gave me a sense of wild abandon. Case in point? I had been wearing my favorite heather-gray DKNY maxiskirt below my belly with a men's white "wife-beater" top. The tank became too small (or I became too big), but I wasn't ready to eighty-six the soft skirt from my fashion repertoire. I yanked it (it had a stretchy waistband) over my engorged boobs and found that I was now in possession of a swingy new trapeze dress. I layered on beads (it was summer) and wore that skirt-as-dress throughout my pregnancy and well into Merry Momdom. This hiked-over-engorged-boobs concept can be applied to any too-tight skirt with an elastic waistband. Examples: A to-the-knee vintage Missoni skirt becomes a festive cocktail frock. A black Lycra miniskirt doubles as a tube top. A maxiskirt becomes a minidress.

Coats as Dresses

The popular designer Kate Spade built her fantabulous retro pregnancy look around cropped jackets and vintage coats (tweed, leopard, woven jacquard) that she wore as dresses. Her trick? Removing the buttons, crossing the garments over in the front, and fastening the fabric with an oversized brooch or two. The kooky brooches were the statement piece. She pulled the look together with tights (often colored), boots or heels, and a colorful bag. NOTE: Coats must be mid-thigh.

Dresses as Tunics

Don't pack up the floaty, easy-to-wear shift dresses of trimester 1 when your stomach balloons. Go with the flow and sport your new dresses-as-tunics with pride. Just add leggings, a ballet flat, wedge, or boot, and you have an entirely new and most functional garment.

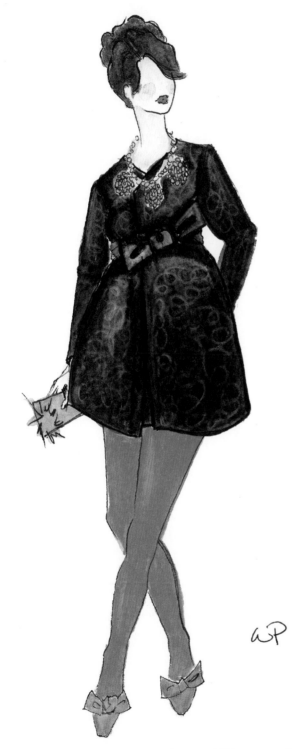

RETRO REDUX A vintage jacket (without buttons) crossed over the chest and tightly belted. This is layered over an empire-waist dress or a skirt worn as a top with skinny (maternity) pants and heels. Shots of color come in the red tights, green purse, and purple shoes. The gold filigree necklace is the Wow Factor statement piece. (Courtesy of Whitney Pozgay for Kate Spade)

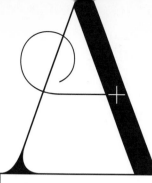

**ADVICE FROM
THE A-LIST**
Jean Godrey-June
Beauty editor, *Lucky*

Lucky magazine was
founded on the premise that
style is about how you put
fashion elements together,
not how much money
you spend. Case in point?
I like the idea of lingerie
as clothing. I wore (and
accessorized) a simple
vintage slip throughout my
pregnancies. People would
stop me and ask—is it
Miu Miu????"

HOT TIP
Flea markets, thrift
stores, swap meets,
and vintage shops are
nightgown nirvana.

Inner Wear as Outerwear

As a fashion editor, I had tons of fancy-shmancy events to
attend while pregnant. One day I was in the tub trying to
cook up something creative for one such event and started
thinking about my grandma Hilda's collection of nightgowns. Going to bed was a ritual for my granny. She took
a fragrant bath, then slipped into a nightie/robe set. Her
nightgowns were no lame Little House on the Prairie redux.
They were Fifth Avenue Fabu, silky, floor-sweeping affairs
emblazoned in racy leopard, tiger, and Pucci prints.
Actually, the nightgowns were not too dissimilar in cut
and fabrication from contemporary ready-to-wear. If top-
drawer designers like, say, Dolce & Gabbana are creating
sexpot collections with gauzy nightgown-like fabric,
then couldn't I wear my granny's nighties to an event?
I mulled it over. A night on the town in a comfy nightgown
was truly the marriage of desire (staying at home and
watching *The Office*) and professional duty. I went for it.
Hilda's leopard nightgown (worn with a boa and Chanel
wedges) was a hit. People kept asking where I got my
of-the-moment maternity dress. Thus began my love of
inner wear as outerwear.

Underpinnings give major look for minor dough.
A bias-cut slip layered with a belted cardigan and funky
jewelry offers *Desperately Seeking Susan* meets *Mrs. Robinson*
cachet. How to get the look? Make a pit stop at your
chic septuagenarian relatives' homes and mine their lingerie
drawers. Nab gauzy nightgowns, caftans, bed jackets,
and slips.

NOTE: *In the forties and fifties, everything was about quality,
so inner wear from this period is often more elegant than
contemporary ready-to-wear.*

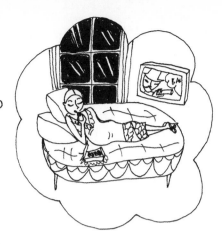

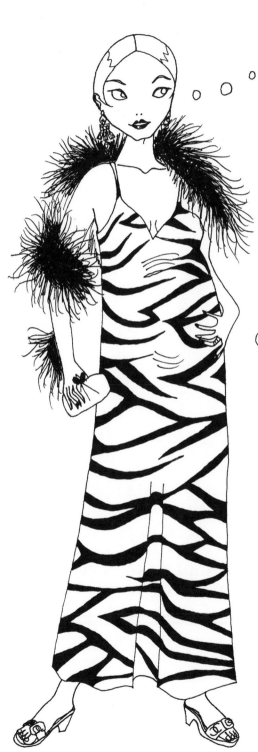

BLOATED
ON THE BIAS

{ **THE BEST OF
BOTH WORLDS**
Out on the town
in a glammy nightie!

How to:
Bump Up a Nightie

Roomy black satin slips make comfy chic dresses. Tie-dyed white nighties make groovy sundresses. Bias-cut long nighties, especially those with interesting swirls of color or prints, make glam cocktail frocks. Little Pucci-esque robes can be belted and worn with a heel. But beware. To avoid the I-just-fell-out-of-bed look, make sure the nightie isn't too transparent. Also, combining lingerie with something more structured like a knit or a jacket adds polish to the look.

Belts as Necklaces

I have a vast collection of thin- to medium-link chain belts that add a Franco-Italianate élan to basic outfits. When these shimmering belts could no longer circle my girth, I popped them over my head and they became flashy Versace-style necklaces. Tie belts can also be worn as lariat necklaces. (See "necklace" in picture on page 108.)

PREGGO PARADISE:
The Swim Department!
The Poor (Wo)man's Versace: Cover-Ups

While we're on the topic of rethinking traditional wardrobe choices, I want to clue you in to the cornucopia of fashion opportunities tucked away with bikinis and sun visors.

I, who detest *la piscine*, am perennially drawn to swimwear shops. A distant cousin of ready-to-wear, swimwear is home to explosively colored, blouson-friendly apparel. Less flashy and far less expensive than ready-to-wear, these no-name bathing-suit "cover-ups" can do double duty as pregnancy apparel. Filene's Basement is filled with tunics that feel like Matthew Williamson and bejeweled linen caftans that smack of Tory Burch. A swirly, candy-colored muumuu I found in Marshall's was a dead ringer for Versace. Macy's groovy animal-print tops echo Robert Cavalli's five-hundred-dollar blousons. Terry-cloth sundresses à la Juicy Couture—you know, the three-hundred-dollar elasticized empire-waist dresses captured in paparazzi shots—are available at swim-wear shops in brandless format for about forty bucks. These whimsical garments have the same jet-set appeal as pricey runway duds at a quarter of the price. Just add leggings, cute sandals, a sea of gold jewelry, and oversized sunglasses.

TIPS ON DRESSING FOR YOUR BODY TYPE

Pregnancy does give you poetic license to dress dramatically. But pregnant or not, a flattering look still hinges upon dressing for your body type—and creating a focal point. Use hem length, décolletage, and garment shape to spotlight your assets. Use accessories to draw the eye to your neck, chest, or arms. Here are some suggestions.

No Butts About It: Bottom Heavy

THINK ABOUT: How to play down the waist and rump and emphasize legs and bust.

TRY: Just-above-the-knee dresses—wrap, shift, empire-waist—that disguise bottom heaviness. Visually elongate the body with a heel. Test-drive pregnancy-specific shapewear to compress your rear and give clothing a smoother appearance. Wear great earrings to bring focus to your face.

NO BUTTS
ABOUT IT

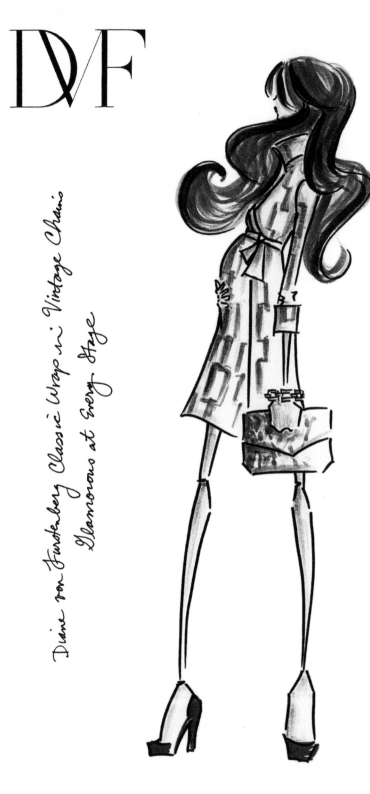

DVF

Diane von Furstenberg Classic Wrap in Vintage Chain Glamorous at Every Stage

{ IT'S A WRAP The easy glamour of a classic Diane von Furstenberg wrap dress with heels is perfect for every stage of pregnancy. The vintage chain motif is super-sophisticated! *(Courtesy of Diane von Furstenburg)*

Thigh Anxiety: Tree-Trunk Legs

THINK ABOUT: Drawing attention up to emphasize your bust, neck, and shoulders. Avoid straight skirts, tapered pants, and pleats.

TRY: Creating a column effect with wider boot-cut jeans and trouser legs that flare slightly at the bottom. Wear full A-line dresses, shirtdresses, and empire-waist dresses. Add a cool scarf or groovy necklace and earrings that play up your glowing face and décolletage. Wear dark colors on the bottom. Test-drive pregnancy-specific shapewear to create balance by compressing your thighs. Wear heels. Ballet flats are too delicate for women with chunky legs.

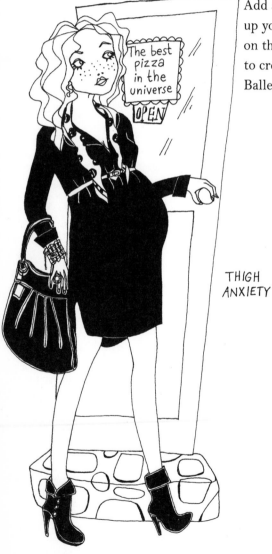

THIGH
ANXIETY

Elongating Your Body:
A Cheat Sheet

- Add verticality with a longer, open cardigan, a dangly long scarf, and/or a flowy shawl.
- Look taller by wearing shorter hemlines (especially important for shorter women) with heels to accent the legs.
- Choose darker colors; they're more slimming.
- Wear an open neckline—V, scoop, or plunging—to slim an explosive bust and give the illusion of a longer neck.
- Make your boots to-the-knee (not calf-length). These will slim and lengthen the leg.
- Opt for longer pants or trousers (that partially cover the shoe) to impart a slimming, vertical line.
- If you're wearing baggy clothing, rein in extra fabric with a belt and/or long layered necklaces for a slimming effect.
- Add height with heels. They not only lengthen the legs but they glamorize most looks.
- Don't forget to point! Pointy toes make you look taller.
- Choose long necklaces to lengthen the torso. Chokers make the neck look short and squat.
- Avoid shiny fabrics. They attract light to all the wrong places, which adds pounds.
- Wear tights that match a dress and boot.

MY BOYFRIEND'S BACK }

Décolletage and a massive dose of legs prove that pregnancy is indeed sexy. The elements: an empire-waist minidress, fishnets, heels, and structured, nipped-at-the-waist boyfriend jacket, proportioned perfectly to make a look that's both flirty and feminine.

(Courtesy of Nanette Lepore)

A mini dress paired with a boyfriend jacket is the perfect look for the pregnant woman. It allows you to show off those sexy legs while lengthening the silhouette

Nanette Lepore

Breast of Luck I: Bountiful Bosom

THINK ABOUT: Reducing the impact of your bust by visually lengthening your torso, neck, and legs. The right neckline makes a big difference. Open, scoop, and V shapes are more flattering than crew or polo necks. The exposed skin breaks up the line from shoulder to chest, minimizing the *kapow* impact of your bodacious boobs. Dark colors on top function as a minimizer. To avoid drawing attention to the chest, stay away from large patterns, light colors, stripes, and adorned tops. Baggy tops will accent the chest and add weight.

TRY: Curve-hugging wrap dresses, empire-waist dresses, or shifts, unadorned tunics, and wider-leg pants to balance proportion. Hems above the knee will draw the eye down. Also, an oversized belt with a gold buckle will draw the attention from your boobs to your belly.

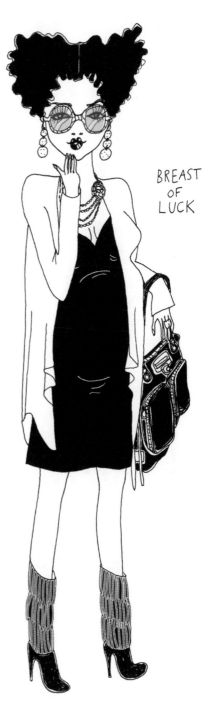

BREAST OF LUCK

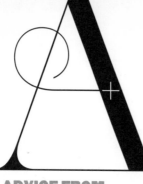

**ADVICE FROM
THE A-LIST**
Kate Spade
Fashion designer

At five feet one, I found pregnancy a balancing act. My trick? I had a uniform and dressed around my bump. I love color. So I bought drawstring skirts in every color from Calypso and wore them as tunic tops. I layered them with a cropped jacket or cardigan tightly cinched with a large Alexis Bittar (vintage-looking) brooch. To streamline the volume on top, I wore maternity cigarette pants and heels. I topped it off with a cool animal-print coat. I also wore a lightweight black jacket as a dress with colored tights. To keep the looks upbeat and fun, I used big rings and flowers in my hair as accents.

Short Stuff: Vertically Challenged

THINK ABOUT: Keeping it skinny on the bottom with a little volume on the top. Scale everything down—fewer adornments, small prints, small pockets—so you're not overpowered by details. Keep all detailing (buttons, stripes) vertical. Avoid baggy clothing. Short necklaces break up the body and can make you feel even shorter.

TRY: Long, lean cardigans make you look taller. Lower-cut shirts give the illusion of a long neck. V-necks lengthen the torso. Keep skirts above the knee. Keep it skinny on the bottom. Pants should be tapered. Flats are okay with a short dress or a cropped pant for summer. Avoid them like the plague during the winter.

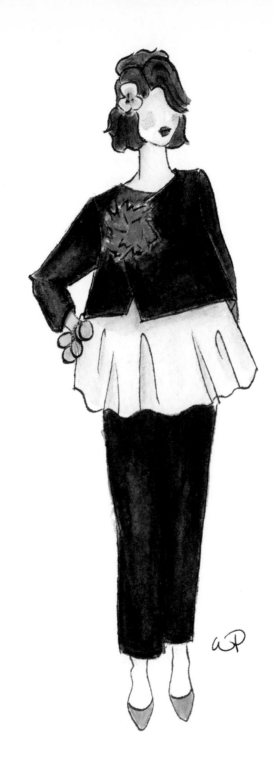

THE GREAT EQUALIZER

Here we have proportion perfection: A swingy trapeze jacket is cinched over a flowy white shirt and worn with skinny pregnancy trousers. The hot-pink floral brooch fastens the jacket and creates a focal point. Lime-green heels elongate the silhouette and add a shot of color. The flower in the hair was Kate's signature accessory. It adds a playful note to the look. (Courtesy of Whitney Pozgay for Kate Spade)

THE SHAPE OF THINGS TO COME: LICENSE TO THRILL

Rotating the basics of your Uniform with Add-ons and Wow Factor is the ticket to effortless pregnancy dressing. And if you wish to stay in this comfort zone, by all means stay put. But your voluptuous state gives you free license to outfit yourself in silhouettes that may never be in your fashion repertoire again. So take advantage of your fecundity with these extraordinarily flattering shapes:

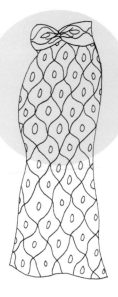

←Hooray for Halters!

The Rolls-Royce of pregnancy shapes, the sensuously cut, tie-around-the-neck halter maximizes boobage and is ultra-flattering to bump-happy babes. Halters come in a shirt and dress form. Add shimmer cream (to cleavage) and some heels for a head-turning ensemble.

←Molto Maxi

The embodiment of bohemian elegance, the floor-dusting maxi is the flowy-chic wonder dress that lets larger women feel feminine and shorter women feel taller. A different pair of shoes and chunky jewelry can take this dress to a casual barbecue or a fancy dinner party. Some tricks: Larger-breasted women need a halter or V neckline; shorter women should have a tightly fitted, empire-waist top.

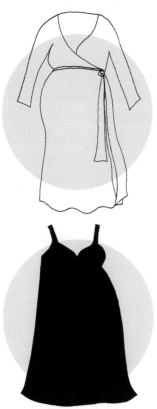

←Wrapper's Delight

The proportion of the clingy fit-and-flare wrap dress is perfection on pregnant women. It hugs your bump, skims your porn-star boobs, slims your torso, and lengthens your legs. The best part? Post-baby, the very same (loosely fitting) wrap dress is a great basic.

←Oh, Baby!

Playful and sweet, the baby-doll dress is perfect for pregnancy.

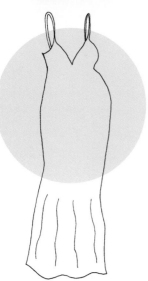

←Be Biased

The bias-cut dress is crafted of diagonally cut fabric that has enough give to hug curves in a sexpot Marilyn Monroe kind of way. Whether it's jersey or satin, the dress has a flow that will enhance a voluptuous, pregnant figure.

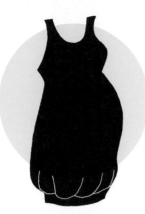

←Blowout

The amorphous bubble dress is a favorite of modern fashion designers. But this tough-to-wear shape can look dumpy on civilians—especially on women with wide hips. But on a woman who's chock-full o' belly, this flirty shape becomes an impressive showcase for the bump. Rein in the excess fabric with a cool under-the-belly belt, and wear slimming opaque tights and boots.

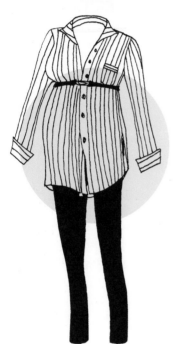

←Flashdance Redux

In civilian life, this leggings look associated with the eighties hit song "Maniac" can be dorky. But in pregnancy, the leggings and boyfriend shirt or sweater look is super-trendy and cute. Add boots and a huge snazzy necklace for up-to-the minute chic.

Some Like It Haute:
My Tailor, My Savior

If you think that a tailor is simply the guy who hems pants, boy, have you been missing the boat. Tailors have the sartorial know-how to make your fantasy ensemble a reality with the flick of a needle. Can't find a dress you like? I couldn't either. So when my bump materialized, I asked my tailor, Boguslaw, to design some gear with me. After ripping out images from fashion magazines, I hit my local fabric store for materials. Boguslaw got to work, and about two weeks later I was the delighted recipient of maternity haute couture: body-hugging bias-cut dresses, floaty trapeze frocks, and colorfully cool jackets inspired by my magazine clippings. (Boguslaw also elasticized the stomach of my favorite non-pregnancy jeans while I was in the between-bloat-and-bulge stage). *Vogue*'s Filipa Fino represents the legions of anti-maternity-clothing-ites who rely upon tailoring as a means to an end. She simply bought regular clothes in bigger sizes and had her tailor nip/tuck them to perfection. She had them altered a second time after the baby was born.

ADVICE FROM THE A-LIST

Alison Brod
Über publicist and all-around trendsetter

For both of my pregnancies I was big on tailoring. So many people make the mistake of wearing clothing that doesn't fit or doesn't flatter their body type. I bought dresses from my favorite stores in a larger size and then, as I lost the weight, had them nipped and tucked minimally to emphasize where I was slimming down. It wasn't cheap, altering outfits a few times, but at least I didn't look like I was wearing a sack every day.

Organization a-Go-Go:
Your Monthly Maternity Checklist

Now that you're really showing, let the list-making begin! If you weren't the planning sort before getting knocked up, you had better fall in love with time frames. There are things to do, outfits to score, a nursery to design and stock, and birthing options to consider. My monthly "to do" list will help you stay on track.

TO DO

Month 4

Photocopy your license and credit cards for when pregnancy brain (see Preggo Glossary) kicks in and you lose your wallet.

TO DO

Month 5

Take a crash course in **Kegels**—the squeeze-and-release pelvic-floor exercises that keep you elastic, you know, down there. If you don't do Kegels, the term "loosey-goosey" takes on a hideous new meaning post-childbirth.

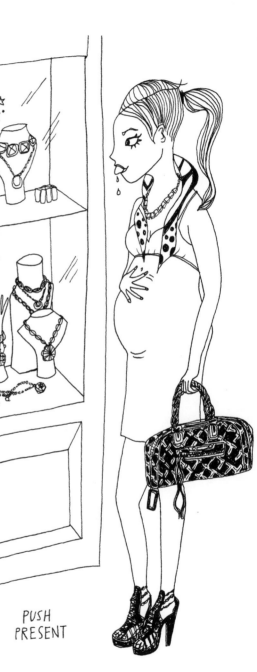

Month 6

Start hunting down your **push present**
(see Preggo Glossary). Get hubby
or partner used to the idea that he may
have to sacrifice his weekly poker nights
(to pool his cash) to honor this age-old
tradition. Fancy jewelry or a fur may
seem excessive. But when you add dollar
signs for each hideous detail of the
pregnancy—nausea, bad skin, cellulite,
huge rump, exhaustion—you rapidly
reach the diamond zone.

PUSH
PRESENT

ACCEPTABLE LOUNGEWEAR: SLINKY VERSUS SWEATS

It's tough waddling about with excess poundage. But unless you're in front of your television, remember that sweats are the enemy. That doesn't mean you have to avoid casual clothing altogether. Simply be selective. There is a huge difference between shlubby sweatpants and sexy, well-fabricated loungewear. Non-maternity brands such as James Perse, Susana Monaco, Ella Moss, American Apparel, Velvet, Clu, Splendid, and Spanx do stylish variations on the legging and yoga pant. On the maternity front, Bella Materna, Japanese Weekend, and Isabella Oliver offer a similar bottom with added belly give.

THE LOOK: PULLING IT ALL TOGETHER
Fashionable (and Foolproof) Fertility Formulas

Glamour is about touches that make an impact. And a dose of confidence. Think about Jackie Kennedy's stunningly simple inauguration ensemble studded with killer earrings and a cape. Audrey Hepburn's oversized sunglasses and brooch-studded coiffure in *Breakfast at Tiffany's*. The Olsen twins' ability to upgrade even a garbage bag with some fabulous vintage trinket. Your charge? Mixing and matching your Adds-ons and Wow Factor accessories to create a cornucopia of haute moderne looks. Here are some formulas that will help you create "looks" while, essentially, repeating the same pieces of your Uniform each week.

- **ABUNDANT ARTISTE** = black V-neck dress + vintage graphic printed duster coat (unbuttoned) + boots + layered tribal beads
- **WEEKEND WARRIOR** = chocolate-brown wrap dress, heavy gold chains, hoop earrings, swirly print tote, black tights, black boots
- **HAUTE GYPSY** = pregnancy jeans + vintage YSL chiffon peasant blouse + open-toe wedge heels + layered gold necklaces and bracelets
- **LA BOHÈME** = black floor-length halter dress + gold flapper-length beads + gold bracelets + gladiator sandals + orange "cozy" sweater

HOT TIP

Snap-happy: When you create a look that you love, snap a photo of yourself in it so that you can easily replicate it.

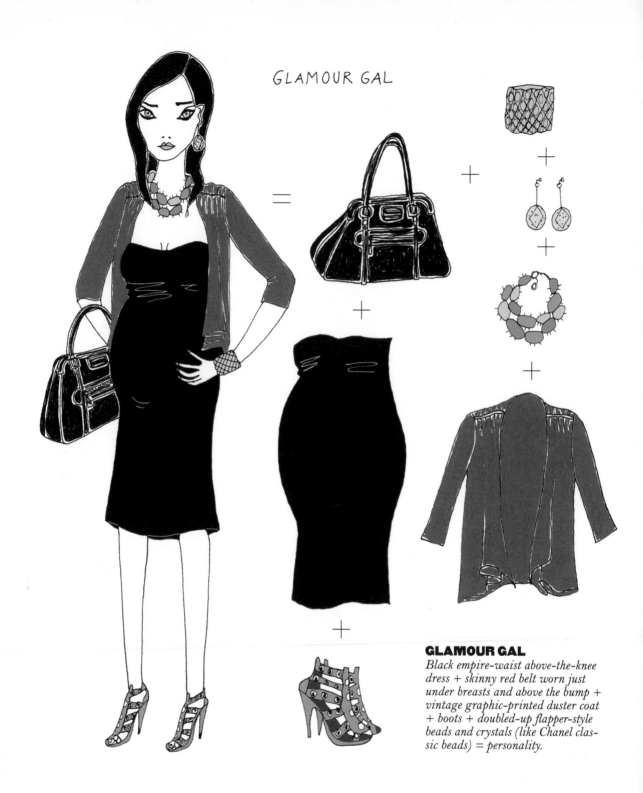

GLAMOUR GAL

GLAMOUR GAL

Black empire-waist above-the-knee dress + skinny red belt worn just under breasts and above the bump + vintage graphic-printed duster coat + boots + doubled-up flapper-style beads and crystals (like Chanel classic beads) = personality.

- **GLAMOUR A-GO-GO** = pregnancy jean + Lycra tank + wide leather grommet belt under the belly + flowy cashmere "cozy" sweater + jeweled gladiator flats
- **LADY WHO LUNCHES** = black V-neck dress + classic Chanel tweed jacket + pearls + stacked-heel pumps
- **PEPPY OFFICE PREGGO** = black pencil skirt + black Lycra tank top + flowy trapeze jacket + black boots with stacked heel + large tote bag
- **NIGHT ON THE TOWN** = black bias-cut dress + crystal-and-gold flapper-length beads + faux-fur shrug or fur boa + fishnet stockings + suede boots with kitten heel + gold-and-crystal evening bag

ADVICE FROM THE A-LIST
Treena Lombardo
Accessories editor, *W*

ON HER UNIFORM
Listen, you can't do maternity in leather. I designed a bohemian look around my glossy Breck Girl hair. Instead of maternity, I bought several sizes of Levis' Type 1 to get me through pregnancy. I bought sack-like dresses (I love designers Marni and Dries Van Noten) in larger sizes, which I super-accessorized with jewelry and shoes. But I also bought loads from H&M, which I now use as beach cover-ups.

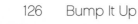

{ **IN-JEANIOUS STYLE**
Citizens of Humanity
pregnancy jeans + slinky
T-shirt + glam accessories
= a Bump It Up Babe.
(Courtesy of Jerome Dahan for
Citizens of Humanity)

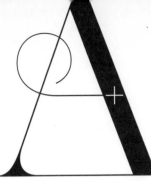

ADVICE FROM THE A-LIST

Wende Zomnir, creative director, Urban Decay Cosmetics

AUTHOR NOTE:
I went through both of my pregnancies with Zomnir and can say with confidence that she is indeed a *Bump It Up* icon.

Nothing says "hot mama" better than a great pair of Citizens of Humanity preggie jeans, a shredded Blondie T-shirt (cut and resewn just the right way to enhance your bump), and some smoky eye makeup with a touch of glitter. The look makes people do a double take and turns you into a conversation piece: "Wow, she's hot! What? She's pregnant?"

Wende's Uniform: pregnancy jeans, Hanes men's undershirts, which she tie-dyed, cropped tees, shrugs, super-form-fitting Michael Stars maternity T-shirts, and reworked rocker tees. Lots of jewelry and huge sunglasses to balance the drama of the bump.

SECOND-TRIMESTER BEAUTY: ON LUMPS, BUMPS, AND UNIBROWS

NONSPECIFIC DERMATITIS

Now that you have (hopefully) conquered first-trimester nausea, up sprouts "nonspecific dermatitis": the code name for a red, flaky rash that, due to hormone fluctuations, often makes a cameo on your face just when your bump shows up. To soothe the skin, look for hypoallergenic, oil-free, non-comedogenic (won't clog pores) products. Cetaphil Gentle Skin Cleanser and Eucerin Redness Relief Daily Perfecting Lotion are the most hydrating and least irritating. For really raw skin and dry flaky patches, rich creams designed for rosacea can work wonders. The compound in B. Kamins Maple Treatment Day Cream and Creamy Cleanser (derived from the sap of Canadian maple trees) is highly effective at softening dry patches and hydrating the skin. You can spot-treat the red areas with an emollient-rich product such as Dermalogica Age Smart Super Rich Repair or Egyptian Magic. If the problem persists, an over-the-counter cortisone cream (always check with your doctor first) applied to affected areas can relieve the itchiness. For itchy skin on the body, soak in a tub filled with Aveeno Soothing Bath Treatment twice a day. You can also add three capfuls of olive oil or almond oil to the bath for increased moisture. Apply cream or essential oils to the body while it is still damp for maximum product absorption. Another trick: Emollient-rich, zinc-oxide-infused diaper cream can be applied to aggravated spots on the face and body to soothe extreme dry skin and calm redness. It is an effective and cheap solution to minor skin irritations. Just remember that it does not soak into the skin, so wipe it off before leaving home!

ACNE

As if you didn't having enough to deal with, raging hormones often trigger minor to severe acne. Elevated progesterone levels (produced by the body during pregnancy to maintain a healthy uterine lining) cause pores to clog, sebum to build up, and oil glands to secrete more oil. What to do? Women with acne should use a mild glycolic cleansing agent (glycol is a natural fruit acid derived from sugarcane) to help the skin slough off dead cells and stimulate regeneration. Aesthetician Sonya Dakar (considered Hollywood's "Fairy Skin Mother" by A-list mamas such as Marcia Gay Harden, Debra Messing, and Gwyneth Paltrow) advises pregnant women with acne to try to have a monthly facial with extractions using a gentle vegetable acid to keep pores open and clear. If you can't get in for a facial, get an all-natural drying mask to kill bacteria and brighten the skin.

BEST BETS: Neutrogena Acne Wash, Sonya Dakar Mud Lavender Mask, Murad Clarifying Cleanser and Clarifying Mask, DDF Blemish Foaming Cleanser, Dr. Hauschka Cleansing Clay Mask.

HOT TIP

The Two O'clock Touch-up: Exhausted pregnant women free-fall after lunch. Perk up at a moment's notice by keeping a stash of beauty minis in your purse or office. Give skin an extra boost with a spritz from a hydrating mister over makeup. Jean Godfrey-June, *Lucky* magazine's beauty director (and total hot mama), has solid advice for pooped-out preggos: "Self tanner and/or bronzer is the ultimate pick-me-up. Use it strategically on face and body as directed, and it will nip the 'you look tired' comment in the bud."

STRETCH MARKS

They are a cruel badge of motherhood. For many women, from the moment they learn of their pregnancy, the fear of stretch marks looms large. Recent studies show that 75 percent of pregnant women are the unhappy recipients of striae gravidarum, reddish scarring that appears where fat is stored: abdomen, breasts, buttocks, and thighs. I hate to be the bearer of bad news, but stretch marks are genetic. If Mom has them, there is a good chance they will show up in your second trimester. And according to the American College of Obstetricians and Gynecologists, research does not support the notion that stretch marks are preventable by the use of creams and stretch-mark-specific oils (though legions of women with a genetic predisposition swear that stretch creams kept them smooth).

But at least you can put up a fight. So says Tanya Mackay of Mama Mio, the London-based maternity skin-care brand. Mama Mio's luxe line is based on hydration through the all-important essential fatty acids. Its Tummy Rub Stretch Mark Oil and Stretch Mark Butter are formulated to replenish and enhance the omegas that the fetus takes during its natural course of development. "To help prevent stretch marks you need to maintain the moisture balance and improve the elasticity of your skin to help it cope with the nine-month stretch," Mackay explains. "If you consume foods rich in omegas and are vigilant about rubbing in moisture—oils rich in omega-3, 6, and 9— throughout your pregnancy, you should be rewarded with your prestretched skin."

Here's what you can do:

- Monitor **WEIGHT GAIN**. Gaining more than the recommended twenty-five to thirty-five pounds increases the chances of developing stretch marks.
- **EXERCISE**: Keeping the blood flowing with exercise boosts circulation and rids the body of toxins.
- Eat **FOODS LOADED WITH VITAMINS A, C, AND E**. Fruits, vegetables, and good fats (olive oil, avocado, salmon, nuts) keep the body hydrated on the inside and maintain skin suppleness.
- **RUB YOUR TUMMY** with a rich cream or oil twice a day. The product should be as pure as possible (chemicals can be absorbed into baby's bloodstream). Look for products rich in omegas, cocoa butter, or neroli oil.

BEST BETS: Mama Mio Tummy Rub Stretch Mark Oil and Stretch Mark Butter, Belli Stretch Mark Minimizing Cream, Nicci Neroli Body Oil, Dr. Hauschka Blackthorn Body Oil, Weleda Pregnancy Body Oil, Bella B Tummy Honey Butter, Basq Resilient Body Oil, organic coconut oil.

ADVICE FROM THE A-LIST
Kim Walls
Founder, Epicuren Baby

Chances are you will develop stretch marks during your pregnancy. Though they are genetic, stretch marks are actually the result of damage to the skin. You can increase tissue resiliency in your body by what you eat. Combat stretch marks by eating foods high in omega-3 essential fatty acids (EFAs) like eggs; fresh, deep-sea fish such as salmon, sardines, and mackerel; borage oil; and flaxseed. Zinc and calcium work with EFAs to help keep the skin soft and lubricated. Excellent sources include eggs, legumes, oysters, spinach, and figs.

A Note on Nutrition:
Tastes Great, Less Lard

To avoid stretch marks and excessive weight gain, limit the carbs. You want pasta and Twinkies; grab the edamame or some nuts. You want fried everything; satisfy your craving to crunch with Pirate's Booty, soy chips, or baked pita chips. Your postpartum body will thank you. Some munchie options: reduced-fat Havarti cheese with grapes; roasted unsalted almonds with dried strawberries or cherries; low-fat frozen yogurt; cherries, kiwis, and mango. Have some of these healthy snacks in your bag so you don't grab junk on the go.

BABYMOON 101

Cruise to Alaska? Jet to Spain? Laze on a tropical beach? Hole up in Michigan? The author's personal research shows that exiting reality and catching up on beauty sleep improves both the complexion and the overall mood of the mom-to-be. From luxurious destination trips to one-day getaways, the travel industry has built an entirely new category of retreat to cater to the swelling (ain't that the truth!) market for expectant parents. The babymoon, a relatively new phenomenon, is defined as that last hurrah, the quiet, so to speak, before the storm. The choices are endless. You can either take a cool trip that does not involve any pregnancy-specific trappings or book a babymoon-branded package complete with features such as goodie bags, in-room prenatal Pilates, and pickles-and-ice-cream-type customization. Some couples simply book a hotel in their hometown for a weekend to luxuriate away from the madness of planning for the new arrival. Excellent options? Las Ventanas al Paraiso in Los Cabos, Mexico, has a babymoon package that comes complete with a director of romance to help plan everything from private-island picnics to exotic couples spa treatments. The "Expecting You" package at the Four Seasons Chicago offers a fantastic goodie bag and weekend filled with in-room massage, manicure, and visits from the ice cream man. The Mandarin Oriental Riviera Maya has a four-day package featuring spa treatments for him and her, private yoga classes, a gift bag, and the pièce de resistance, a blessing from a Mayan medicine man. For less pricey options, B and Bs are getting in on the game, offering cozy weekend retreats with extras such as in-room massage, non-boozy bubbly, and a keepsake box for baby. Keep in mind that obstetricians don't like you to fly after the seven-month mark, so plan early. Try www.baby-moon.eu, www.babymoonguide.com, or www.bnbfinder.com/babymoon for listings.

Dos & Don'ts:
Finessing the Incredible Bulk

DO

- Invest in a multitasking V-neck **BLACK DRESS**.
- Let your bump guide your fashion choices by sporting the kind of **GROOVY GARMENTS** that you would choose in your civilian state—for example, a maxidress, a halter dress, a baby-doll.
- Wear **BIG ACCESSORIES** (especially a huge tote bag) to match the bravado of your bump.
- Buy fabric and have your tailor **RE-CREATE** your favorite dresses in larger sizes.
- Showcase your **CLEAVAGE** at every opportunity.
- Wear **FISHNETS**.
- Wear pregnancy **SHAPEWEAR** to hold everything in.
- Look to accessories to **PULL A LOOK TOGETHER**.
- Invest in **SHIMMER** and **BRONZER**.

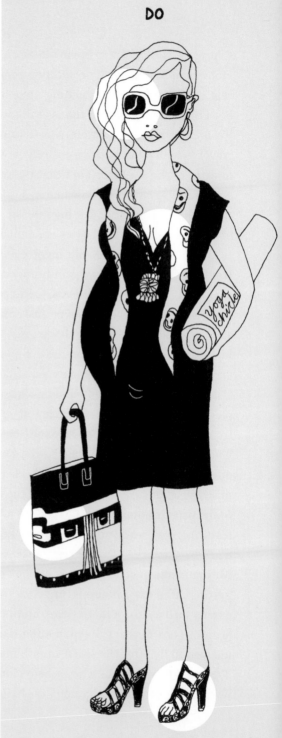

DO

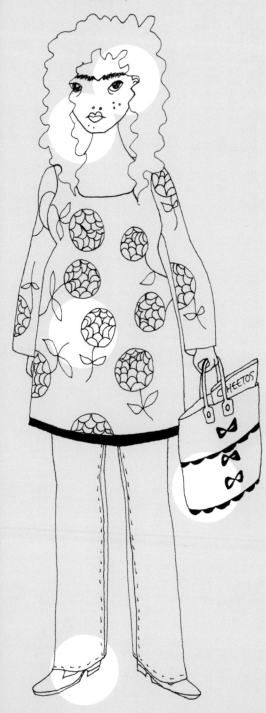

DON'T

DON'T

- Wear frumpifying **CALF-LENGTH** dresses.
- Trade your chic hobo bag for a scuzzy Cheetos-filled **SACK**.
- Wear **SENSIBLE SHOES**—frumpola!
- Think your **INNER RADIANCE** negates the need for makeup.
- Say **GOODBYE TO YOUR HAIR COLORIST**. Most hair dyes are completely safe during pregnancy.
- **STOP EXERCISING**.
- Eat large quantities of **SALT**. You will swell. Everywhere.

Large and In Charge

Nothing frumps you up
like . . . a dumpy purse . . .
horizontal stripes . . . a matronly
coat . . . a below-the-knee
dress . . . round-toe shoes . . .
(too-small-bra-induced)
back fat . . . a beige outfit . . .
scruffy nail . . . lack of
accessories . . .

You are showing and (hopefully) glowing big-time. You've mastered garment rotation, gotten a doctorate in dramatic accents, and become fluent in the language of accessories. You have a penchant for prints and know how to work pops of color into a minimalist wardrobe. **Volume control is second nature.** With your massive belly taking center stage, you need to revel in your fecundity. Step 1? Punch up the Wow Factor to match the bravado of your bump. Wear ten bracelets instead of five. Buy peacock-feather earrings. Add an extra Liberace-style cocktail ring. Try animal-print pumps. Use an even bigger tote in an electric color. Put a brooch in your hair.

Another fun way to punch up third-trimester zing is through makeup. My friend Wende Zomnir, founder and creative director of the edgy Urban Decay makeup brand, crafted a sexy "I ain't your average preggo" smoky eye to draw even more attention to her fecund frame. And when you're drained by all of the diva-like drama surrounding you, R & R awaits in the form of pregnancy-specific pampering.

PUTTING ON THE GLITZ

Your large and in charge stature gives you the ability to do the unexpected. Ask yourself, WWCBD (What would Carrie Bradshaw do)? And dress accordingly. This means lots and lots of accessories so you can simply rotate your uniform(s) day in and day out.

GLOBAL GODDESS

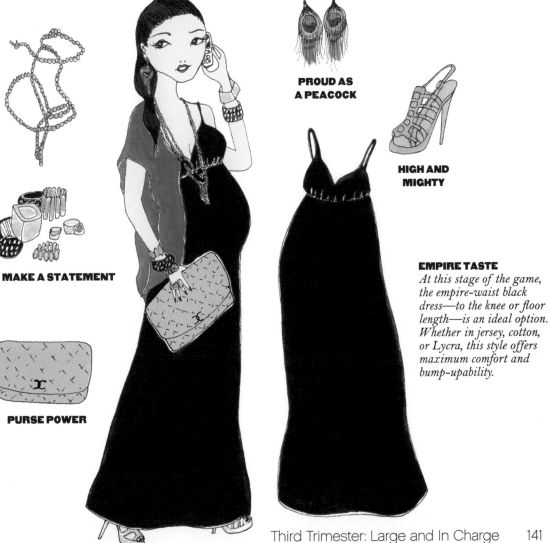

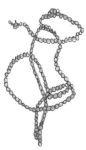

MAKE A STATEMENT

PURSE POWER

PROUD AS A PEACOCK

HIGH AND MIGHTY

EMPIRE TASTE
At this stage of the game, the empire-waist black dress—to the knee or floor length—is an ideal option. Whether in jersey, cotton, or Lycra, this style offers maximum comfort and bump-upability.

BLACK-TIE SOIRÉE WHILE
IN THE FAMILY WAY

There are times during pregnancy when one must go beyond the average basic. Case in point? The black-tie soirée. Should such an invitation materialize, you can test-drive the nightie-as-evening-wear look. If luxed-up lingerie is not your speed, elegance can be delivered in the form of the floor-length low-cut empire-waist dress. Here's why: The open neckline draws attention to the décolletage, the shoulders, and the arms (often unscathed by pregnancy weight gain); the just-under-the-bust waistline provides cascading fabric that falls loosely over the bulging butt and bump; and the floor length is fancy and flattering because it elongates the figure. This enduring silhouette is offered season after season and can be found at maternity and non-maternity shops at every price point.

Drawing attention to the décolletage with a beaded strap and open neckline while minimizing the baby bump with a pleated tulle tier is a sexy and elegant way to do evening –

A dramatic accessory like a mink stole adds a needed soupçon of glamour.

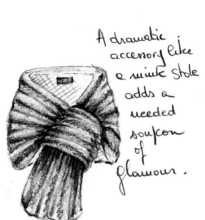

the three-tier silhouette has an elongating effect and the pale color is incredibly sophisticated.

Mendel 08

{ **EVENING ELAN** A red-carpet favorite, J. Mendel is all about transforming a basic silhouette into the realm of high art. Here, another head-turning approach to the floor-length empire-waist dress. Gilles Mendel offers his signature glamour with a three-tiered pleated tulle gown with beaded straps. The design minimizes the bump and elongates the figure. P.S. Dangly earrings add a dramatic dimension to this look. (Courtesy of Gilles Mendel)

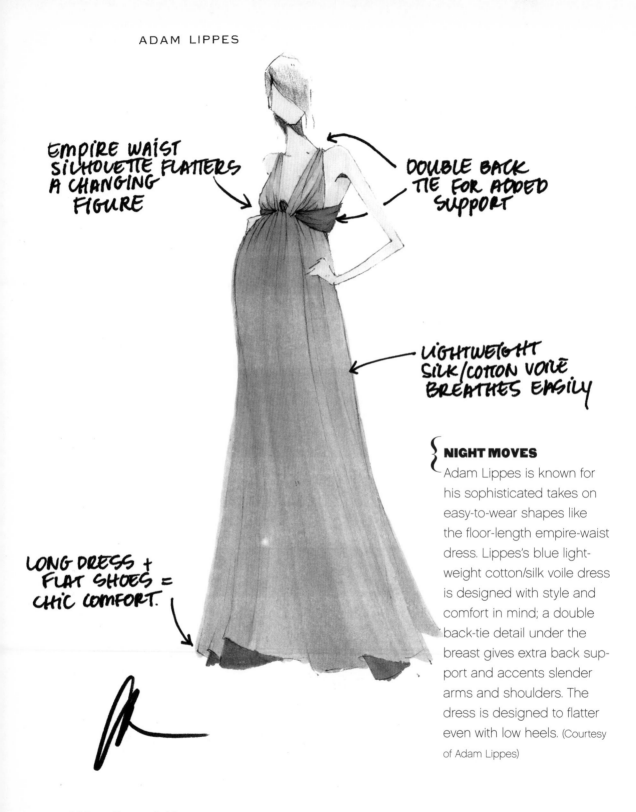

EMPIRE WAIST
SILHOUETTE FLATTERS
A CHANGING
FIGURE

DOUBLE BACK
TIE FOR ADDED
SUPPORT

LIGHTWEIGHT
SILK/COTTON VOILE
BREATHES EASILY

LONG DRESS +
FLAT SHOES =
CHIC COMFORT.

NIGHT MOVES

Adam Lippes is known for his sophisticated takes on easy-to-wear shapes like the floor-length empire-waist dress. Lippes's blue lightweight cotton/silk voile dress is designed with style and comfort in mind; a double back-tie detail under the breast gives extra back support and accents slender arms and shoulders. The dress is designed to flatter even with low heels. (Courtesy of Adam Lippes)

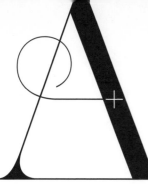

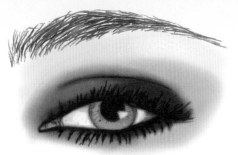

(Courtesy of Wende Zomnir for Urban Decay)

ADVICE FROM THE A-LIST
Wende Zomnir, creative director, Urban Decay Cosmetics

THE SMOKY EYE

Fortunately, there's an easy way to smoke out your eyes that looks classy, cool, and just a bit dangerous. The most important rule is that smoky eyes involve only a little bit of black. Raccoon eyes happen when the black is a little too free-flowing—bad on any girl, worse on a pregnant woman. So here goes . . . there seem to be a lot of steps, but they're just baby steps that make smoky eyes easy to execute.

1. Pick a shadow shade that enhances your eye color.

2. Pick a coordinating eye pencil (I recommend Urban Decay's long-lasting 24/7 pencils): gray (Gunmetal), plum (1999), green (Stash), or taupe (Underground).

3. Get yourself a long-wearing black pencil such as 24/7 in Zero, and promise yourself to use it sparingly.

4. Apply an eye-shadow primer. You want your look to last all day, and pregnant-lady-with-creased-and-smudged-shadow is not a good look.

5. Grab a matte, nude shadow and apply from the crease to the top of your brow bone. Apply a tiny bit of matte white shadow along the arch of your brow to add some dimension.

6. With your finger, smudge your selected shadow shade all along your upper lid and right into the crease. Use a crease brush (shaped like a pointed paintbrush) to blend the shade to just above the crease, making sure the colors mesh seamlessly.

7. With a little brush, smudge a little shadow all along the rim of the lower lashes.

8. Line both upper and lower lash lines all the way around with your coordinating eye pencil. Make the line thicker

at the outer corner of the upper lashes. Make it soft, and blend it into the shadow.

9. Now get out that black pencil and sharpen it to a fine point. Line the outer fourth of the lower lash line. Using your little brush, smudge the black on the lower lashes into the pencil and shadow. Leave the upper lash line fairly sharp.

10. This part gets tricky, but it's essential for a smoky eye, and it's important to use a long-lasting black pencil. Line the inner lid of the upper lash line. Hopefully, your pencil has a softer point on it now. Don't tug at your eye. Just look straight ahead and line. It's a little unnerving the first time, but it adds so much intensity that you won't want to skip it.

11. Apply lots of mascara.

Dos and Don'ts: Mastering Maternity Moxie

DO

* **WEAR BLACK**, black, and more black.
* Wear a **ZANY MAXIDRESS**.
* **GET DRAMATIC** with a smoky eye.
* Treat yourself to a day (or a week) at the **SPA**.
* **TAKE A PHOTO** of yourself in various forms of undress so you can whip them out ten years down the road.
* Hop in the **POOL**—a pregnant body is weightless when swimming.
* Concoct a **BIRTH PLAN**.

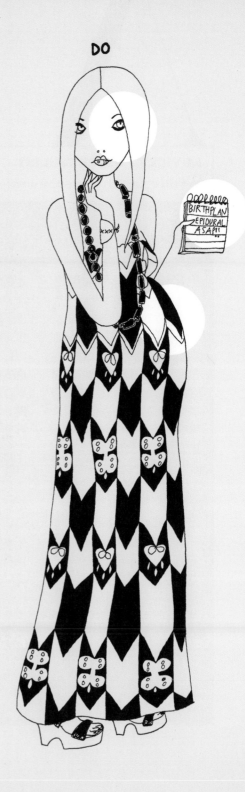

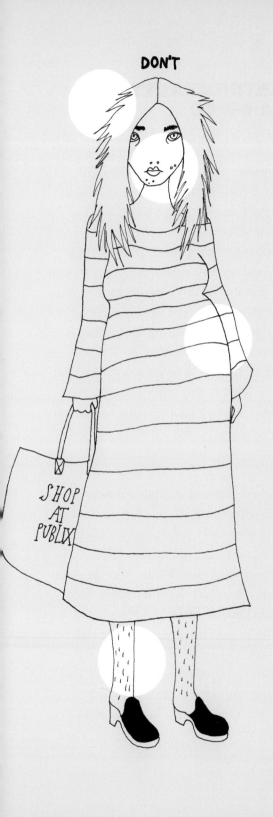

DON'T

DON'T

* Give in to "feeling like crap" by sporting jumbo clothing and **SACK DRESSES**.
* Wear anything with **HORIZONTAL STRIPES**.
* **FORGET TO MAINTAIN** your grooming regimen: brows, bikini, mani/pedi.
* Allow anyone with garlic breath or dirty fingernails to **TOUCH YOUR BELLY**.
* **OBSESS** about how you will lose all of this weight.
* Let anyone get into the third sentence of a **CHILDBIRTH HORROR STORY**.
* Show up for the birth looking like a cavewoman with **MATTED HAIR** and **BUSHY BROWS**.

THIRD-TRIMESTER BEAUTY: PAMPERING A-GO-GO

Voluptuous. Abundant. Teeming with Life. During the third trimester, feeling glamorous has everything to do with pampering. There are two reasons that you should revel in your procreative state. Pregnancy is tough work, and you deserve a massive dose of self-indulgence. The other reason is that your life is about to change for good. Did you notice, perchance, at your baby shower how every single gift was for the baby, not you? You, the star of this baby-making production, are being subtly notified that a new boss is entering the house. FYI, this bizarre put-on-the-back-burner feeling is an indicator of your new life as provider and mom. The moment that child is born, the focus will turn from you to your newborn. Unsettling, no? That is why you absolutely must spend these last few weeks treating yourself like a superstar.

GET THEE TO A SPA

In the past decade, spas have witnessed explosive demand for pregnancy-specific treatments. With so many contra-indications involved with pregnancy (no hot tub or sauna, no massaging certain points of the feet, no contraband ingredients that could harm the fetus), women wanted—no, demanded—rejuvenating treatments that they knew were safe. In response, day spas have developed bodywork and facials that strictly adhere to guidelines put forth by the American College of Obstetricians and Gynecologists. Indulging in prenatal massage is relaxing, true. It will also help to assuage the ligament aches, leg pain, and lower back strain of the last trimester. Facials (no contraindicated ingredients or too-active peels) during pregnancy are an excellent way to ward off melasma, encourage cellular turnover, and eliminate the toxin buildup that impedes the coveted pregnancy glow.

Whether you live in Miami or Mundelein, Illinois, booking a safe spa treatment is a snap. Many top-tier hotels, including the Mandarin Oriental, the Four Seasons, and Peninsula, offer prenatal services at all of their properties. At all sixteen Bliss Spa locations (most are inside W Hotels; go to www.blissworld.com for locations) "maxed-out moms-to-be" can sign on for Great Expectations, a seventy-five-minute prenatal massage to relieve "tired muscles, tension, swelling, overstretched and itchy skin, and sluggish circulation." Internationally acclaimed skin-care brand Mama Mio took its "no nasties" policy to the next level by developing Mama's Touch Maternity Spa Treatments, catering to the needs of moms-to-be. Upscale properties such as the Ritz-Carlton and Canyon Ranch offer the Mellow Mama maternity massage, the Lighten Up foot soak, and the Smoothie exfoliating facial using Mama Mio products. Perhaps the largest variety of services is available at Edamame Maternity Spas (a division of Destination Maternity), which cater only to pregnant women (there are seven locations that can be found on www.destinationmaternity.com). Weight gain and swelling are taken on with massage. The Vital Leg Treatment reduces water retention and increases circulation to fatigued legs and feet. And a series of facials addresses uneven skin tone, oiliness, and/or dehydration.

HOT TIP

To find a destination or day spa near you, use the excellent resource www.spafinder.com. Simply plug in your zip code and "prenatal services," and a listing will come up. For spas offering Mama Mio's Mama's Touch services, visit www.mamamio.com/us/finals/spa1a.html.

DIY PAMPERING

If you can't get to a spa, there is no shortage of ways to nurture yourself. Create little treats to look forward to: a pedicure on Fridays, a nightly foot massage with an awesome-smelling cream, a sexy pout-plumping lip gloss. Turn your bathroom into a sanctuary with candles. Hop into a warm bathtub into which you've added some almond oil and a few drops of lavender essential oil. Put on a soothing facial mask and chill out. Then have your husband or partner massage your aching body, cramped feet, and painful pelvis. There are scores of articles and videos on how to do pregnancy massage online. He owes you, no?

DELIV-A-CHIC: READY, GET SET, WAX!

I don't care what your friends have told you. The final month of pregnancy is not for counting contractions over a tray of Fannie May Mint Melt-Aways. Month 9 is all about preparation to look thoroughly divine in the delivery room. With the proliferation of Skype, YouTube, and Facebook, all the world's a stage. Even the birthing room. Do you

HOT TIP

Weight gain, shifting posture, and ligament stretching put enormous pressure on the lower back, knees, and legs. Not to mention your aching feet. Prenatal massage alleviates back pain and is both relaxing and supremely therapeutic for moms-to-be.

want your gorgeous new baby overshadowed by your talons, unibrow, and frizzy tresses? Delivery pics will be posted moments after the cord is cut and sent to your online address book. Then Mom, Grandma, sister, and in-laws will get to work forwarding images to your friends, colleagues, and every last acquaintance until your sleepover-camp bunk mate (whose bed you short-sheeted) ends the cycle. Since your image will live in perpetuity on the World Wide Web, a month 9 rendezvous with your glam squad is essential. I made the mistake of canceling my brow appointment the week before delivery of my first child and had disastrous results. My daughter Isabella was beautiful. But my unibrow usurped her radiance, giving the whole birthing scene an unwelcome *Planet of the Apes* vibe. Treat your delivery like a paparazzi-encrusted outing, and groom accordingly.

Grooming Checklist

- Keep your **BROWS** groomed. Nothing looks and feels more glam than perfectly manicured brows. Remember the words of the sagacious brow queen Anastasia: "Everyone in Hollywood knows that great brows make your hips look smaller!"
- Have a **BRAZILIAN WAX**. After two kids and extensive research, I can say with confidence that doctors and nurses appreciate a shrub-free zone.
- Get a **MANI** and **PEDI**. Beautifully polished hands and feet just make you feel better.
- Keep your **HAIR** styled. Due dates are never a sure thing, so be prepared by scheduling a blowout each week leading up to D Day.
- Keep **MAKEUP**—especially blush and under-eye concealer—on hand to freshen up frazzled features after an arduous delivery.

Organization a-Go-Go:
Your Monthly Maternity Checklist

WHAT TO PACK FOR THE HOSPITAL

A due date is an educated guess. To be completely prepared for D Day, have your hospital bag packed and ready by week 32. It will give you a semblance of order and control. Consider your needs: The room will be freezing and dry. The food will be gross. There will be no Ritz-Carlton amenities in the bathroom. And you might be there longer than you think. Make your quarters and yourself comfortable with little touches from home. A cozy cashmere shawl or blanket is soothing for the hours of labor you may endure. Thick socks are a must. Your feet will be exposed in the stirrups and can get really cold. A robe that smells like home for the day after delivery is comforting. Have a great-smelling cream on hand for after the delivery; it will feel great and minimize the antiseptic smell of the hospital. Make a delivery-specific playlist for your iPod or burn a few CDs with your favorite chill-out music. It's fun to be able to remember the exact song that was playing when you gave birth. A nice neutral lip gloss instantly prettifies a tired postpartum visage.

YOUR BAG SHOULD CONTAIN:

- A printed **LIST OF WHO TO CALL** from the hospital with big news. If you want to e-mail pics, have e-mail addresses already loaded into your computer.
- A cozy cashmere **SHAWL** or **BLANKET** from home to snuggle in during the early stages of labor and after delivery. Delivery rooms are freezing.
- Bottled **WATER** and **SNACKS** for post-delivery.
- **TOOTSIE POPS** help with delivery. You cannot eat or drink once delivery starts, so a few sucks in between contractions supply the body with enough sugar to keep pushing.
- **MAKEUP**.
- **LIP BALM**.
- **MOISTURIZER** for your face and body. Did I mention that the room is super-dry?
- Make two **CDS**, one for each stage of delivery: dilation and delivery. Ambient yoga music and soft-rock for dilation and classic rock for pushing.
- **CAMERA**.
- **GRANNY UNDIES** (to house the diaperlike pads you will be sporting on the drive home).
- Loose **OUTFIT** to wear home.
- **LAYETTE** (see Preggo Glossary).
- **GIFTS** for your nurses. They work hard and really appreciate the gesture.

Month 7

Head off on your last relaxing **trip** before baby. Sleep late, have sex, and enjoy your last flight without schlepping a car seat and diaper bag. Take a sexy pregnancy photo in an exotic locale.

Month 8

Investigate pediatric experts and buy their books. **Read** and highlight information about feeding, sleeping, burping, and colic so you're not quasi-informed when you bring the baby home.

Month 9

Get a blank journal and create a **color-coded log** to chart baby's first month. Sleep, diaper changes, and feeding time should be recorded in order to get him or her on a schedule.

HOT TIP

Leave the G-string at home! You will require granny undies or your husband's tightie whities to secure the diaper-like pads you'll wear for weeks after delivering. With my first delivery, I was clueless and had the embarrassing task of asking my father-in-law to head out and buy me briefs.

NESTING 101

In the last stages of pregnancy, your desire for cheese is matched by a craving to edit the household and get everything ready for baby. This is the world-famous "nesting" instinct. Go with it. Having your home systematically organized will supply you with order in the face of the forthcoming chaos.

- Set up the crib, changing table, and rocking chair/gliding chair in the **BABY'S ROOM**.
- Buy all of the creams, lotions, medicines, and miscellaneous **ITEMS FOR THE NURSERY** (see "The List" on p. 160).
- Buy **CLEAR PLASTIC CONTAINERS** and organize baby clothing, accessories, and toys.
- Buy a label maker to **ORGANIZE CLOTHING** in plastic bins— 3–6 months, 6–12—so garments can be easily organized and accessed.
- Have **CARPETS** steam-cleaned.
- **ORGANIZE KITCHEN CABINETS** and drawers and make room for bottles, bibs, pacifiers, et cetera.
- Throw out your **OLD MAKEUP**.
- Clean out your **LINEN CLOSET**.
- **SHINE** tarnished jewelry and picture frames.
- Make a **"BIRTHING" PLAYLIST** on your iPod.
- Program the hospital **TO-CALL LIST** on your cell phone, and make an extra chip for your husband.
- Make **FILES** for photos, doctors, travel plans, insurance, and other important things in your life.

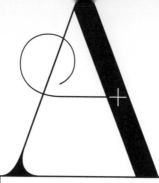

Susan Harmsworth, CEO and founder, ESPA

For puffiness around the ankles and legs, soak feet in cool water with Epsom salts added, and while your feet are immersed, apply cool eye pads to help reduce puffiness and revitalize the eyes. In fact, an Epsom salt bath will help swelling anywhere in your body as well as relieving aches and pains. Just be sure to keep the bathwater lukewarm and drink cool water while in the tub. To ease tired, aching legs, follow with an application of a cooling balm to reduce fluid retention, then elevate the legs and relax (try to elevate your legs as much as possible during pregnancy, and also drink lots of water, as you can easily get dehydrated).

A simple way to elevate the legs is to raise the leg end of your bed a few centimeters (an old book under each leg will do). An age-old remedy for swollen legs is the daily ritual of skin brushing with a firm-bristled body brush. Begin at the feet and very lightly sweep upward toward the bikini line. Repeat this on the front and back of the legs twice daily for a more severe case of swollen legs, once daily for slightly swollen legs.

PUSH IT TO THE LIMIT: SOME DELIVERY TRUISMS

Though this is a style book, I am including some facts that I wish had been revealed to me prior to labor and delivery. What the female body can endure is mind-boggling and beautiful. And delivering a baby is one of the most empowering experiences in life. But it also hurts like hell and in no way resembles that cheeseball *Great Expectations* movie that is shown in hospitals when you get the labor and delivery tour.

Here are a few facts—graphic but true—that may help you:

- If you go into labor naturally, you may have the slow, steady ebb and flow of cramps that lead to full-fledged contractions à la the *Great Expectations* movie shown in your birthing class. Or, like me, you go into stage 4 right off the bat. Contractions feel like someone has taken Emeril's steak knife and is slashing each and every corner of your back to shreds. Be prepared.
- You may experience what I call "contractive Tourette's syndrome." This is normal. I don't curse much, but once my contractions started, I became a potty-mouthed pig. If this happens to you, know that the nurses have seen everything. Just apologize in between contractions and continue your rant.
- Don't be afraid to ask for an epidural immediately. In fact, I told my doctor when I was five months pregnant that I was no martyr and would like to be drugged at the one-centimeter-dilation mark. Get this in writing, as your doctor may not be on call when you go into labor. The nurses always tell you to wait. Fuggeddaboutit. Nip that pain right in the bud. And, so you know, the epidural is the easy part.
- Side effects from the epidural (about ten minutes after the injection) are shivering and itching. The discomfort is manageable but unnerving if you don't know what to expect.

- After the epidural is administered, the agony of the contractions is blocked, allowing you to actually doze off until you're dilated enough to deliver. But don't get too excited. The epidural is turned down super-low when it's time to push so you can feel the contractions and "push through."
- With an epidural, you lose all feeling from the waist down, so you cannot get up from the delivery table. Because you cannot get up, a catheter is used. When it is removed and you pee for the first time on your own, there is a lot of blood. And what they call "matter." It is totally normal but can be pretty scary stuff if nobody informed you about it.
- Pushing is really hard work. It means holding in your abdominal muscles and bearing down as if you are making a huge poop. You feel as if you should be standing. But with an epidural, you have to birth lying down. The squeeze-and-release pelvic-floor contractions of Pilates are excellent practice for pushing.
- Pooping on the table is normal and happens to most women. Don't stress out about it.
- If you tear or have an episiotomy, the first few poops after the baby feel as if you have sat on a smoldering fire. Make sure that your nurse gives you stool softener after the delivery. Enough said.
- Though you have a birth plan, you never know what will happen. Women who want a natural birth with a doula or midwife may need an epidural. Your vaginal birth may have to go C-section because of the baby's position. Be open-minded if your plans go awry. A healthy baby is the most important thing.
- Make your decision about breast-feeding before you go into labor. If you decide to breast-feed, they will hand you the baby (after cleaning him up, of course) right away to get going. If not, they will clean up the baby and you can give him the first bottle.

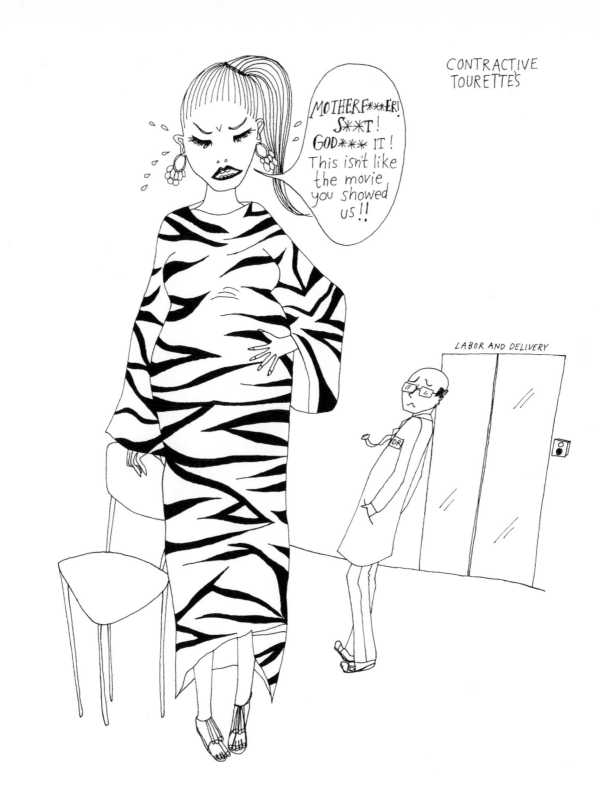

THE LIST: MUST-HAVE GEAR FOR THE NURSERY

- ☐ A + D Original ointment
- ☐ Aquaphor Baby
- ☐ Baby bathtub
- ☐ Baby bottles (Dr. Brown's Natural Flow [BPA-free] are my favorite)
- ☐ Baby carrier (Baby Björn is my favorite)
- ☐ Baby mittens (to keep baby from scratching herself)
- ☐ Baby monitor
- ☐ Baby swing
- ☐ Baby-grooming kit: nose suction, nail clippers
- ☐ Band-Aids
- ☐ Bibs
- ☐ Bouncy seat
- ☐ Burp cloths
- ☐ Car seat (Britax is my favorite)
- ☐ Diaper bag
- ☐ Diaper Genie or other odor-free receptacle for dirty diapers
- ☐ Diapers
- ☐ First-aid kit
- ☐ Formula
- ☐ Fragrance-free/dye-free detergent such as Dreft
- ☐ Hot/Cold Boo Boo Pack (for bumps and bruises)

- ☐ Infants' acetaminophen
- ☐ Liner for changing table
- ☐ Multi-use pads for bassinet
- ☐ Mylicon Gas Relief drops or gripe water
- ☐ Organic baby body wash
- ☐ Pacifiers
- ☐ Pedialyte
- ☐ Q-tips
- ☐ Receiving blankets
- ☐ Snap-N-Go or fold-down stroller for car
- ☐ White-noise machine (if you live in a noisy environment)
- ☐ Wipes

FOR THOSE BREASTFEEDING

- ☐ Breast milk storage bags
- ☐ Breast pump
- ☐ Lansinoh Nipple Cream
- ☐ LilyPadz reusable nursing pads

NEWS FLASH: No alcohol, powder, or creams on newborns. And no baths until the umbilical cord has completely fallen off and the belly button has healed.

Lighten Up!

Nothing frumps you up
like ... baring your spare
tire of a tummy ...
breast-milk stains ... a cutesy
headband ... matte
lipstick ... a mid-calf skirt ...
bad sunglasses ...

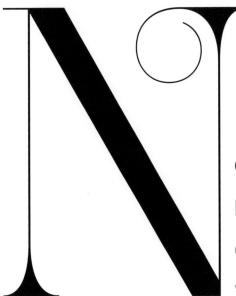ow that you have your bundle of joy, it's time to start focusing on how to deal with the other bundle, your postpartum bod. When you come out of the birthing haze and glance down at your deflated beach ball of a stomach, you can't help but curse your Cinnabon intake and think, "Christ! How am I going to lose this freakin' flab??" It's awkward. You aren't pregnant but your pre-preggo clothes still look like they belong in the closet of a dollhouse. A week after I had my first baby (I was en route to an emergency brow plucking after seeing how my unibrow marred delivery pictures) an acquaintance smiled at me and innocently inquired, "When is the baby due?"

I thought about hosing the offender with breast milk. But reality is reality. Since it took nine months to get this large, it would take some time to shrink back to my gamine frame. Actually, the fourth trimester, or transition trimester, is about "lightening up" across the board: losing weight, evening out skin tone, and not being too hard on yourself.

TRANSITION CLOTHING

AT YOUR LEISURE

By the time you have your baby, you are tired. Tired of
being pregnant. Tired of eating. Tired of being kicked in
the ribs all night. Tired of peeing every fourteen minutes.
And tired of your preggo wardrobe. Sorry, but you will
need to stick it out for another few weeks. We all fantasize
about leaving the hospital in our pre-pregnancy jeans,
just a wee bit swollen and slightly the worse for wear.
But a baby only weighs about seven pounds. And the fluids
about ten pounds. The rest is baby-induced blubber. You
don't have much to worry about for the first week or
so because you will probably not leave your house. The
beginning of motherhood is nothing short of boot camp
with high-pitched hunger shrieks as your reveille. Pee on
the changing table! Poop! Barf! Bottle! Pump! Outfit
change! Is she sleeping? How long will she sleep? Do you
think he's hungry? How can I get this kid to burp? Should
we call the doctor? Honey, is he breathing?? With chaos
and new demands consuming your day, the object is to be
comfortable in nonbinding clothing. While you're bonding
with baby at home, sport comfy loungewear that can withstand puke stains: leggings, soft, roll-down yoga pants, cool,
breezy caftans, shirtdresses, and cotton T-shirt dresses.

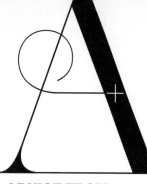

**ADVICE FROM
THE A-LIST**

Aliza Licht
VP, global PR, Donna Karan

After the baby, I wore a
Donna Karan Body Perfect
toner/shaper under every-
thing. It is a seamless boy
short that is a modern-day
girdle. During my maternity
leave, I stayed in my jersey
maternity dresses. They
are forgiving and the most
flattering option.

STEPPING OUT: CAMOUFLAGE CLOTHING REDUX

Unless Heidi Klum's personal trainer has been making house calls to you, there is no way that you'll be able to squeeze into your pre-preggo clothing for quite some time. Why? Your hips are still splayed in childbearing position. Your butt and thighs are clinging to the daily enchiladas. And, oh yeah, you just had a baby!!! To transition your still-bloated bod back into civilian clothes, it's all about mind over matter. Approach the situation knowing that "this" (grab fistful of flesh on stomach) is all water weight with a dash of bagel. You will get back to your old slinky clothing. You will! Tweak your drapey pieces and do not waste money on garbing this temporary shape. With exercise and a healthy diet, your body will morph back to its pre-pregnancy shape. Save your cash for Manolos. And Pampers.

The fourth trimester is pretty similar to the first. You simply don't want to look fat. The problem this time around is that you have much more weight to camouflage. Again, you have a choice: you can give in to your exhaustion and walk around looking like an extra from the set of *Lost*, or you can step up to the fashion plate and pull yourself together. Move away from form-fitting, bump-kissing duds and head back to drapey, nonstructured shifts, trapeze dresses, tunics, and empire-waist camouflage clothing. Once again, rely on these body-skimming silhouettes (see pages 10–12) to strategically cover the pooch and conceal your porn-star breasts. If it's winter, love thy sweater and shirtdress. For spring/summer, make nice with empire-waist sundresses, slip dresses, or a simple A-line. Continue to think about volume and proportion. Showing décolleté with V-necks, scoop necks, and low-cut tops will elongate the torso. Add length with a heel. The tricks outlined earlier—empire waisting, long, layered necklaces, verticality, and open nonstructured knits—will extend your silhouette and draw attention away from the midriff. The only purchase you should make is a pair of "transition" jeans. After a few weeks of running around like a lunatic, you will have lost some water weight and will be able to retire your pregnancy jeans for civilian denim (two to three sizes larger than your pre-pregnancy size). With the help of a belly band, these should work for about three months.

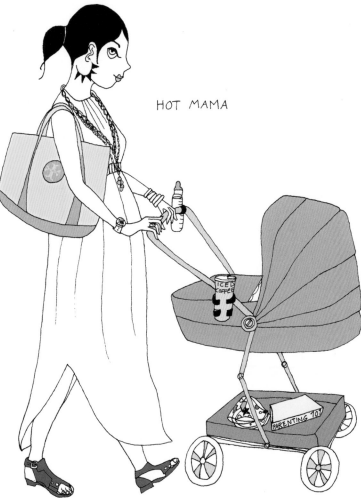

HOT MAMA

FOURTH-TRIMESTER LOOKS

- Preggo jeans or transition jeans with tunic top
- Black empire-waist dress with scarf or shawl creating verticality and coverage of postpartum pooch
- Stretch-cotton-jersey dress with scarf or shawl creating verticality and coverage of postpartum pooch
- Shift, slip dress, or shirtdress with a long, open-knit cardigan
- Soft cotton T-shirt dress and leggings
- White button-down and leggings

How to:
Coolify Ill-Fitting Transition Jeans

The transition jeans that you buy will fit in the waist, hips, and butt but be pretty roomy in the legs. To eliminate the hand-me-down look, customize them. Cut the too-long hem and fray it with sandpaper. When you wash the jeans, they will emerge with a tattered hemline à la Marc Jacobs. Wear the jeans below the hipbone for a slouchy/boyfriend look. Use your belly band. It will be like rediscovering an old friend on Facebook.

SLIMMING CLOTHING: YOUR MAIN SQUEEZE

Recently, inner-wear companies had a brainstorm. Noting celebrities' addiction to shape wear on the red carpet plus a spike in "leisure wear" sales, they decided to incorporate these two trends into one revolutionary garment: shape-wear-enhanced leisure wear! Perfect for the fourth trimester, these pieces offer chill-out clothing with built-in compression technology that slims while you slave. Donna Karan Body Perfect's Waist Embrace Capri is a slimming legging that can also be worn as inner wear. Belly Bandit offers the Mother Tucker compression tank top (with anti–roll up technology) and Yummie Tummie's hip-length or long-length slim-wear camis mask muffin-top flubber when you wear skirts and jeans. And the Spanx Bod-a-Bing! skirt and cropped pant (only available on spanx.com) are both equipped with a built-in liner for a smoother, firmer look.

BREAST OF LUCK II: BREAST-FEEDING

Breast-feeding adds another element to getting dressed. If you are breast-feeding, remember to insert nursing pads into your bra. Proof of the super-cool connection existing between you and your baby is evidenced in the fact that milk comes spurting out each time the baby cries. It also leaks when it's time to pump. Just be prepared. It's a good idea to stick to darker-color tops until you become adept at gauging leakage.

If you're not breast-feeding, you need to bind your breasts until the milk dries up. If you don't start breast-feeding at the hospital, it takes about a day or two for your milk to come in. After my baby was born, I was watching a rerun of *Sex and the City* when, between the opening credits and the girls being screwed over by whatever guy was featured on that episode, I morphed into Pamela Anderson. Having decided not to breast-feed, I bound my aching breasts in an Ace bandage and then put a skintight jogging bra over it. A more stylish approach to breast binding is the Bosom Bandit, a six-inch support wrap (lined with cooling gel), which supports engorged breasts while suppressing lactation. To help with swelling, a frozen bag of peas on each breast molded perfectly. I layered this becoming getup under everything (even my nightgown) until the milk dried up. Another pointer: If you want your milk to dry up, do not let your breasts get wet in the shower. Any type of stimulation, especially warm water, will cause milk to come gushing out, thus undermining your efforts.

MUST-HAVE POSTPARTUM ACCESSORIES

1. DONNA KARAN BODY PERFECT WAIST EMBRACE MID-THIGH SHAPER is a silky second skin that reduces the appearance of postpartum lumps from below the bra line to mid-thigh.

2. LILYPADZ (www.lilypadz.com) are the revolutionary alternatives to disposable nursing pads. These silicone rubber pads have a tacky lining that adheres to the nipple and stops breast-milk leakage. They are reusable and, unlike traditional lumpy pads, look smooth under clothing. You can use them whether you are breast-feeding or not.

3. A RUBBER DOUGHNUT: If your episiotomy left your nether regions looking and feeling like chopped sirloin, get yourself a rubber doughnut for comfortable sitting. Grab a Sharpie pen and fancify this hideous cushion by drawing interlocking C's (à la Maison Chanel) directly on the rubber. Plop it right down on the restaurant chair (are chairs always this hard?), and watch passersby ogle your would-be luxury apparatus with covetous curiosity.

4. **SEAMLESS HIPSTER UNDIES**: Jockey's microfiber Comfies underwear is an inner-wear dream for the new mom. They are wide enough to accommodate the postpartum pads, sleek enough to wear under dresses, and super-comfortable because they're thin and stretchy. Many brands make seamless microfiber undies, but the Jockeys are inexpensive, so when you stain them, you don't have the same heart-wrenching reaction that comes with the loss of your "good" panties.

5. **A SHAPEWEAR CAMI**: Layered under tops or worn alone, the genius microfiber technology compresses postpartum pudge.

THE MIRACLE OF SHAPEWEAR

As soon as you're on your feet, immediately redirect all food cravings into a shapewear obsession. A niche category of hosiery, shape wear is the stealth bomber of postpartum dressing. These microfiber bulge busters can whittle your waist, trim your thighs, lift your rump, and slim your entire midsection. Shapers are essentially modern-day girdles that compress excess body flab to deliver a sleeker you. But shapewear has a secondary function. The abdominal compression helps to decrease uterine swelling and the bloating caused by water retention. In essence, the faux whittled waist will yield a true whittled waist.

Brands such as Jockey, Flexees, Soma, Maidenform, Sassybax, Yummie Tummie, and Miraclesuit make shapers with varying degrees of compression. Immediately after pregnancy a stretch microfiber high-waist-to-mid-thigh undergarment like Spanx's Power Panties, the silky Donna

HOT TIP
When a relative or friend asks if you need anything, tell them that the ultimate gift would be a steak dinner and a body shaper.

Karan Body Perfect Waist Embrace, Maidenform's Control It! High-Waist Thigh Slimmer, or Lipo in a Box's High Waist capri can sleekify your silhouette and smooth the appearance of postpartum lumps. Squash muffin tops with shapewear camis from Yummie Tummie, Sassybax, Belly Bandit, or Spanx. For maximum postpartum compression, try Donna Karan Body Perfect's Body Toner unitard, which extends from spaghetti straps to just below the knees to squeeze you into too-tight clothing. If your bulging tummy is the only concern, try Maidenform's Control It! Brief or Nancy Ganz Tumm-EE-Breef for support. The wonderful site www. shapewear.com is a resource for tips and brands to suit every body type. Barenecessities.com carries most brands mentioned here.

LIGHTEN UP! HOW TO GET YOUR BODY BACK

In terms of weight loss, don't expect much in the first two weeks. Little by little, your abdomen contracts and your rib cage starts sidling back to its original home. As you begin to move around more and eat well, your metabolism will fire up and you will naturally burn through some of the pregnancy blubber. Losing the baby weight is similar to parenting. The keys are to anticipate needs and be prepared to divide and conquer.

BYE-BYE BLUBBER

The first step to losing weight is obvious. Throw away all of the junk food in your house and replace it with fruits, steamed vegetables, proteins, grains, and yogurt. Ask your parents and in-laws to bring over healthy foods so you have them on hand when hunger strikes. In exchange for their generosity, load them up with all of the fattening "treats" people drop off to celebrate the birth of the baby. Here's the catch-22 about post-pregnancy weight loss. Food is the last thing you want as you stare at that spare tire dropping over your jeans. But eating is required to bolster your metabolism. High protein, fruits, and whole grains boost energy and burn calories. Instead of eating three big meals, have four to five small meals per day so you keep your metabolism fired up. Stop eating by 7 P.M. Frequent meals keeps your blood sugar steady so you don't fall victim to binge eating. Also, keep healthy snacks—whole wheat crackers, dried figs, carrots, and fruit—in your purse so you don't succumb to junk-food pit stops.

To speed up the loss of water weight, drink fennel tea and squeeze lemon in your beverages. Fennel is a diuretic that helps you knock out water weight and flush toxins. Lemon (a key ingredient of Stanley Burroughs's infamous Master Cleanse) is another diuretic that helps the body eliminate water weight and toxins. FYI, seltzer and lemon is a great way to curb the appetite until it's time for your next meal.

HOT TIP
Fennel and lemon are natural diuretics that flush toxins and knock out water weight.

REFLEX-OLOGY

Now, to knock out snacking, you have to get Pavlovian. So how do you go from downing an entire key lime pie to just craving the lime? It's simple. Imagine that the green pie with whipped cream and extra-crunchy crust is a fetid mass of raw sewage. That's right. You must come up with a repulsive visual that helps you deny the urge to suck down whatever caloric treat is in your path. Self-imposed environmental conditioning, or what I call the postpartum Pavlov effect, involves retraining your mind's reflex to see the stimulus, an unhealthy carb or sweet, as a "gross" versus a "yum." Sounds depraved, but this tried-and-true technique has worked successfully for supermodels and actresses.

I am not suggesting starving yourself. Just cutting the crap. Literally.

YOU GOT TO MOVE IT, MOVE IT

Bolstering the metabolism is also a matter of exercise. You should not do any strenuous exercise until the doctor gives you the go-ahead at your six-week checkup. But you certainly can increase your activity after two weeks by taking your baby out for walks and beginning light toning movements. Be realistic. If you stayed in shape during your pregnancy, you will have the endurance to work out more quickly after the baby is born. Fred DeVito, creator of Exhale Spa's butt-kicking Core Fusion workout, aided me and hundreds of postpartum women in losing baby weight. "Look at any and all movement as exercise," he advises. "The more physical you are, the faster you will establish a physical lifestyle and focus on getting yourself back in shape." Translation? Take power walks around the neighborhood with your baby. Pay homage to Studio 54 by blasting disco and dancing with your newborn around the house. Put the changing table on the second floor so you have to go up and down the stairs many times a day. At the six-week mark, start getting back to an exercise regime. An amazing at-home workout can be had with Fred DeVito and Exhale's DVDs Core Fusion Pilates Plus and Core Fusio: Body Sculpt. Or hit a gym that offers child care. It's amazing how the baby fat literally melts away after a few months of vigilant exercise.

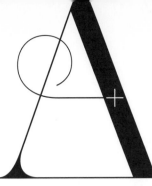

ON JUMP-STARTING THE METABOLISM

In the first six weeks after delivery, prior to working on your core muscles, you can turn your focus to your thighs and butt. By strengthening and toning these two large muscle groups, you can raise your overall metabolic rate, which in turn speeds up your ability to burn calories and drop weight.

THIGH STRENGTHENER

Stand with your feet hip-width apart and parallel. Keeping your knee straight, raise your left leg to the height of your hip and then touch the toe to the floor, twenty times. After twenty, keep your leg hip high and do three sets of twenty small lifts. Hold the last one, and raise both arms up above your shoulders for five seconds, then release. Repeat with the right leg.

BUTT STRENGTHENER

Lie on your front in plank position with elbows bent and forehead resting on top of wrists. With both legs straight, hip-width apart, pull abdominal muscles in and drop your tailbone. Keeping your knee-caps facing straight down or parallel, lift the straight left leg off of the floor without allowing the left hip to rise from the floor. Do two sets of twenty. Then bend the left knee and lift the thigh off of the floor for two sets of twenty. Next, keeping the left knee bent, turn the left leg out from the hip (meaning the kneecap no longer faces down, it faces slightly left, depending on your degree of turn-out). Do two sets of twenty lifts. Then, keeping the leg turned out, go back to a straight left leg and finish with two more sets of twenty straight leg lifts. Try to keep the left knee off the floor through the transitions. Repeat the entire four-part sequence on the right side.

NOTE: No sit-ups or crunches until you are six weeks postpartum.

CELLULITE, CELLULITE, WHERE AIN'T MY CELLULITE?

My pal Aliza Licht had another great strategy to stop eating junk food. She intentionally wore skintight spandex at home during her maternity leave in order to maximize the impact of her postpartum bulges. "I looked hideous," she explains. "Staring at the layers of flab hanging over my pants inspired me to do all of the right things to lose weight." Of course, she did not wear spandex out of the house, preferring seasonless jersey maternity dresses. "I was back into some of my pre-pregnancy clothes within two months." I took a similar approach. I would stand nude in front of the mirror each morning to make sure that I stayed the course of eating well and exercising. Again, sounds perverse. But it works.

ABDOMINAL COMPRESSION

For centuries, women from all walks of life have relied upon abdominal compression, or "belly binding," to flatten and tighten postpartum tummies. Wearing a compression garment for six to eight weeks after childbirth helps reduce uterine swelling and bloating. This, in turn, speeds up the redefinition of a waistline. Recently, a new mom torqued this age-old concept into a high-style postpartum tool: the Belly Bandit (www.bellybandit.com/). And celebs such as Angelina Jolie, Gwen Stefani, and Halle Berry are raving about it. It comes in five sizes and three styles (I love leopard!). A less expensive approach is to bind your tummy with a good old Ace bandage.

FOURTH-TRIMESTER BEAUTY: SALVAGING YOUR SKIN

Thanks to skyrocketing hormones and chronic exhaustion, your face probably reads like a pregnancy diary: Melasma from the summer by the lake. Spider angiomas (burst blood vessels) on the side of your nose from pushing. Under-eye puffiness from lack of sleep. And a smattering of acne from general toxicity. The upside of the fourth trimester is that, after nine months of scrutinizing every ingredient that you slather on your body, you can once again indulge in hard-core skin-care regimens (but check the ingredients with your health care practitioner if you're breast-feeding). To quote Dr. Harold Lancer, "Skin is the ultimate accessory." Tapping into the right products and treatments will recharge your complexion.

HYPERPIGMENTATION

One of the biggest issues for women of all ethnicities is pregnancy mask or hyperpigmentation. Hyperpigmentation takes time to reverse. If you haven't been exfoliating throughout your pregnancy (tsk!), now is the time to get a home scrub such as Dr. Brandt Microdermabrasion Exfoliating Face Cream, Epicuren Micro-Derm Exfoliating Cream, Philosophy's Microdelivery Peel, or Olay's Regenerist Thermal Skin Polisher. Sloughing off the dead, damaged skin and stimulating new cell growth is a critical component of evening out the skin tone. Exfoliating three times per week will enhance the skin's ability to absorb lightening creams and other topical products. Remember: Exfoliation + lightening products = even skin tone.

STEP 1: To even out the skin tone, use a lightening mask (Epicuren Skin Lightener, Kate Somerville Clearing Mask, Sonya Dakar Lightening Mask), which contains naturally occurring bleaching agents. These products can reduce facial discoloration by inhibiting tyrosinase, the enzyme that causes hyperpigmentation. Apply the mask only to the dark area for the first six weeks, then to the whole face to even out the skin tone. Best bets contain one or more of the following ingredients: kojic acid, hydraquinone, glycolic acid, lactic acid, licorice, and Japanese mulberry.

STEP 2: Use a night cream or serum with retinoids (Skin-Ceuticals Retinol 0.5 and Neutrogena Ageless Intensives Tone Correcting Concentrated Serum) in conjunction with a moisturizer to lighten and brighten the skin. For sensitive skin, dermatologists recommend Kinerase, which is specifically formulated with kinetin for photo-damaged and retinoid-intolerant skin. Also for sensitive skin, Skin-Ceuticals' Phyto Corrective Gel is a skin-lightening agent that uses botanicals in place of hydroquinone, a bleaching agent. If discoloration persists, Dr. Lisa Airan recommends Tri-Luma, a prescription-strength triple-action steroid cream containing fluocinolone, tretinoin, topical vitamin A, and hydroquinone. "The hydroquinone in Tri-Luma decreases the formation of melanin (which causes dark spots) and will reduce or eliminate dark spots within eight weeks," she explains. *NOTE: If you are breast-feeding, you must avoid products containing retinoids.*

SPIDER VEINS

Until recently, women were forced to camouflage unsightly spider "angiomas" with mountains of concealer. Not anymore. The FDA-approved Lyra Laser zaps targeted blood vessels in seconds. There is no topical product to treat spider veins.

DEHYDRATED SKIN

After delivery, it's time to tackle dull, dry skin with a more aggressive skin-care regimen. Antiaging products are your gateway to luminosity. Upgrade your skin care with creams, masks, and serums rife with nutrients that combat free radicals, slough off dead cells, and stimulate the synthesis of collagen, a prerequisite for healthy, glowing skin. The latest and greatest potions exfoliate and hydrate with active ingredients; antioxidants, proteins, vitamins, peptides, lipids, essential acids, and minerals. Here are some of my favorite products to revive the complexion.

ANTIAGING PRODUCTS: THE GATEWAY TO LUMINOSITY

To Brighten Sallow Skin

BEST BET ESPA Super Active Skin Brightening Enzyme Mask: A high concentration of active ingredients (marine bio actives, phyto-active compounds, and essential oils) exfoliates skin, leaving you looking bright-eyed and refreshed. Available at Peninsula Hotels and www.espaonline.com.

To Treat Fine Lines and Wrinkles

BEST BET A "cocktail" of Kate Somerville Quench and Deep Tissue Repair: Hyaluronic acid, layered with peptides and omegas, locks in moisture and makes skin velvety and younger-looking. Available at Sephora and www.katesomerville.com.

To Hydrate Seriously Dry Skin While Treating Fine Lines and Wrinkles

BEST BET A "cocktail" of Sonya Dakar's Cellular Patch Cream and Omega-3 Repair Complex: Layering the plant-derived omega-3 and omega-6 fatty acids, green tea extracts, and pure apricot kernel and sweet almond oil improves dehydration, skin clarity, and firmness without irritation. Available at www.sonyadakar.com.

To Calm Inflammation, Hydrate, and Replace Essential Fatty Acids

BEST BET Kinara Intense Peptide Serum: Hefty doses of ceramides and essential fatty acids in ingredients such as kukui nut oil and evening primrose oil soothe very dry skin and improve skin texture. Available at www.kinaraspa.com.

LASER AND LIGHTS: THE FASTEST WAY TO REJUVENATE POSTPARTUM SKIN

Hyperpigmentation and the visible signs of pregnancy stress (exhaustion!) take time to reverse with products. If you are type A and want immediate results, you can whip distressed skin back into shape with topical of-the-moment procedures. Noted laser treatments are topical and, aside from the Mixto, have zero downtime. And yes, they are expensive.

Intense Pulsed Light (IPL)/ Photorejuvenation

For hyperpigmentation, intense pulsed light treatments destroy dark spots with heat while stimulating healthy new collagen formation. Here's how it works. The skin is numbed and a machine held close to the face delivers sequential pulses to the targeted area without damaging surrounding skin. The next day the pigmentation rises like scum to the surface of your skin; it flakes off a few days later. IPL also smooths skin and decreases fine lines and wrinkles.

LED Rejuvenating Facials

For her A-list clientele, Kate Somerville recommends a series of facials with LED (light-emitting diodes) to cleanse, stimulate, tone, and refine. This topical treatment (offered by medi-spas around the country) involves a shield like a *Star Wars* helmet that hovers over the face delivering low-level light therapy. The light activates fibroblasts and regenerates tissue, allowing dry skin to retain moisture, a prerequisite for dewiness.

Titan Laser Treatments

Tighter, younger-looking skin can also be had with the Titan laser. Titan is the first nonsurgical light-based system approved by the FDA for the safe treatment of lax skin of the face, neck, and body. An infrared-light source tightens skin and reverses the signs of aging by stimulating long-term collagen rebuilding. The Titan works by delivering heat into the deeper levels of the skin's tissue, causing the collagen to tighten and contract. It's safe, painless, and a great alternative to more invasive procedures. Titan is also being used to help postpartum bellies bounce back. The recommended course is approximately three treatments, spaced four to six weeks apart, over the course of three to four months.

Chemical Peels

Dr. Lisa Airan has her postpartum patients go through a series of chemical peels to reclaim radiant skin. A chemical solution (glycolic, lactic, or salicylic acid) is applied to face, neck, and décolleté, creating a surface wound to activate the body's healing response. Dry, damaged skin literally peels off. This treatment helps reduce spots and wrinkles.

CO_2 Laser Resurfacing

For serious hyperpigmentation, Airan is a fan of the new fractionated MiXto laser, which "resurfaces" dull and damaged skin. A CO_2 beam comes in direct contact with the epidermis, heating and vaporizing the tissue, which evenly treats damaged areas. The entire complexion temporarily darkens, and within three days the discoloration flakes off. The laser tightens the jawline, de-puffs the eyes, smooths the skin, and thoroughly evens out the skin tone. Because it speeds up collagen production, the effects of two or more treatments are cumulative. There is about one week of downtime (you'll want to stay home, as your face will be quite red).

KEEPING IT ALL TOGETHER

When your belly explodes into a regulation-sized NCAA basketball (consequently making the contents of your closet resemble the sales floor of American Girl Place), a fashion freakout is indeed in order. But you took the reins and mustered mega-maternity moxie. By retooling your approach to fashion you succeeded in using your bump to triumph over frump. And in the process, you did not waste your unborn child's college tuition on a full-blown wardrobe with a short shelf life.

In no time you will be back to your sveltissimo self and all of your pre-pregnancy accoutrements. The *Bump It Up* philosophy served you well in pregnancy. But I have a secret to share. Although you no longer need to dress around the bump, the tenets of garment rotation can still help you in your new life as a mom. As you resuscitate your pre-preggo wardrobe, keep it well edited and organized. The concept of a foolproof Uniform enhanced by Add-ons and Wow Factor is the key to effortless dressing. So when things get chaotic, draw upon your nine-month crash course in glamour. Basics are blah unless you bump them up!

ACKNOWLEDGMENTS

I want to get down on my knees and kiss the Manolos of Debra Goldstein, my fantabulous agent at the Creative Culture. She is the X to my Y, with her unflagging support yielding our child, *Bump It Up*.

A huge shout-out to Pamela Cannon, Porscha Burke, and the rest of the stellar team at Ballantine/Random House. Thanks for "getting" me and helping me focus and organize the many, many components of this book.

Thank you to all of the incredible designers, beauty wizards, and all-around style hounds who contributed to this book: Rachel Roy, Donna Karan and DKNY, Isaac Mizrahi, Tim Quinn, Maria Cornejo, Michelle Smith, Rafe Totengco, Nicole Miller, Devi Kroell, Stacey Bendet, Kate Spade, Nanette Lepore, Diane von Furstenberg, Adam Lippes, Gilles Mendel, Wende Zomnir, Jerome Dehan, Simon Doonan, Cojo, Kate Somerville, Sonya Dakar, Dr. Harold Lancer, Dr. Lisa Airan, Jen Rade, Fred Devito, Cameron Silver, Gabby Reece, Aliza Licht, Filipa Fino, Jean Godfrey-June, Treena Lombardo, Rae Ann Herman, Alison Brod, Mara Stern, Jill Kargman, and Kim Walls.

Thanks to my inhumanly patient husband, Peter, for his support and countless explanations to our children that mommy's book was what made her so crabby.

Finally, a hearty thanks to my dearly departed artiste grandmother Hilda Koch, my style icon, who insisted that forty-two bracelets, four necklaces, and a few knuckle-duster rings always "worked" with my look.

RESOURCES

Fashion

Adam Lippes: www.shopadam.com
American Apparel: www.americanapparel.com
Balenciaga: www.balenciaga.com
Barneys New York: www.barneys.com
Betsey Johnson: www.betseyjohnson.com
Calypso: www.calypso-celle.com
Chanel: www.chanel.com
Citizens of Humanity: www.citizensofhumanity.com
Clu: www.shopstyle.com
Comme Des Garçons: Barneys New York
Diane von Furstenberg: www.dvf.com
DKNY: www.dkny.com and Bloomingdale's
Dolce and Gabbana: www.dolceandgabbana.com
Dries Von Noten: Barneys New York, Blake in Chicago, Jeffrey in New York and Atlanta, Maxfield in L.A., Stanley Korshak in Dallas
Ella Moss: www.ellamoss.com
Fogal: www.fogal.com
Hermès: www.hermes.com
Isaac Mizrahi: www.isaacmizrahi.com and www.lizclaiborne.com
Issey Miyake: Saks Fifth Avenue and Issey Miyake stores in New York
James Perse: www.jamesperse.com
J. Mendel: www.jmendel.com
Kate Spade: www.katespade.com
Levis: www.levis.com
Marc Jacobs: www.marcjacobs.com and Bloomingdale's
Marni: www.marni.com
Matthew Williamson: www.matthewwilliamson.com
Milly: www.millyny.com and Nordstrom and Bloomingdale's
Missoni: www.missoni.com and www.netaporter.com, as well as Curve in L.A., Jeffrey in New York, Blake in Chicago, and Barneys New York
Nanette Lepore: www.nanettelepore.com

Nicole Miller: www.nicolemiller.com
Rachel Pally: www.rachelpally.com
Roberto Cavalli: www.robertocavalli.com
Splendid Clothing: www.shopbop.com and Nordstrom
Susana Monaco: www.susanamonaco.com
Tory Burch: www.toryburch.com
Urban Outfitters: www.urbanoutfitters.com
Van Cleef & Arpels: www.vancleef-arpels.com
Velvet: www.shopbop.com
Versace: www.versace.com
Vince: www.vince.com
Wolford: www.wolford.com and department stores
Yohji Yamamoto: upscale department stores and specialty shops
YSL: www.ysl.com
Zero + Maria Cornejo: www.zeromariacornejo.com

Maternity

Belly Dance Maternity: www.bellydancematernity.com
Boing Boing: www.boingboingmaternity.com
Cadeau: www.cadeaumaternity.com
Due Maternity: www.duematernity.com
Ingrid & Isabel: www.ingridandisabel.com
Isabella Oliver: www.isabellaoliver.com
Krista K: www.kristak.com
L'Avenue des Rêves: (212) 396-9500
Liz Lange: www.lizlange.com
Mommy Chic: www.mommychic.com
Motherhood Maternity: www.motherhood.com
Mylo Dweck Maternity: (718) 333-0420
A Pea in the Pod/Destination Maternity: www.apeainthepod.com
Pickles & Ice Cream: www.picklesandicecream.com
Rosie Pope: rosiepopematernity.com
Veronique Maternity: www.veroniquematernity.com

Lingerie/Shapewear

Bella Materna: www.bellamaterna.com
The Belly Bandit: www.thebellybandit.com
Donna Karan Body Perfect: department stores
  nationwide
Fertile Mind: www.fertilemind.com
Flexees: www.maidenform.com and Macy's and Kohl's
Hanro: www.hanro.com
Japanese Weekend: www.japaneseweekend.com
Jockey: www.jockey.com
Lilyette: www.maidenform.com and Macy's and JCPenney
Lipo in a Box: www.lipoinabox.com
Loving Comfort: www.lovingcomfort.com
Maidenform: www.maidenform.com
Medela: www.medela.com
Miraclesuit: www.miraclesuit.com
Nancy Ganz: www.bodynancyganz.com
Natori: www.natori.com
Sassybax: www.sassybax.com
Soma: www.soma.com
Spanx/Assets: www.spanx.com and Bloomingdale's
  and Nordstrom
Wacoal: www.wacoal-america.com
Yummie Tummie: www.yummietummie.com

"Fast Fashion"

Bebe: www.bebe.com
H&M: www.hm.com/us
Topshop: www.topshop.com
Zara: www.zara.com

Vintage Stores

CHICAGO
Lulu's at the Belle Kay: www.lulusbellekay.com

LOS ANGELES
Decades: www.decadesinc.com
Lily et Cie: 9044 Burton Way, Beverly Hills
  (310) 724–5757
Resurrection Vintage L.A.:
  www.resurrectionvintage.com

Sielian's Vintage Apparel:
  www.sieliansvintageapparel.com
The Way We Wore: www.thewaywewore.com

MIAMI
CMadeleine's: www.cmadeleines.com
Fly Boutique: www.flyboutiquevintage.com

NEW YORK
The Dressing Room Bar and Boutique:
  www.thedressingroomnyc.com
Chelsea Girl Couture/Laurel Canyon Vintage:
  www.chelsea-girl.com
  (212) 343–7090
Edith Machinist: 104 Rivington St., New York
  (212) 979–9992
The Family Jewels: 130 West 23rd St., New York
  (212) 633–6020
Resurrection Vintage New York:
  www.resurrectionvintage.com
What Goes Around Comes Around:
  www.whatgoesaroundnyc.com

Online Vintage Resources

eBay: www.ebay.com
enokiworld: www.enokiworld.com
Etsy: www.etsy.com
Marion Mercer: www.marionmercer.com
Monster Vintage: www.monstervintage.com
Rusty Zipper: www.rustyzipper.com
TheFROCK: www.thefrock.com
Vintage Vixen: www.vintagevixen.com

Beauty

Avalon Organics: www.wholefoodsmarket.com
Aveeno: drugstores nationwide
Basq: www.basqnyc.com and Neiman Marcus and
  Saks Fifth Avenue
Bella B: www.destinationmaternity.com
B Kamins: www.bkamins.com
Bobbi Brown: www.bobbibrowncosmetics.com
Burt's Bees: www.wholefoodsmarket.com
Cetaphil: drugstores nationwide
DDF: www.ddfskincare.com
Decleor: www.decleordirect.com

Dermalogica: www.dermalogica.com
Dr. Brandt: www.drbrandtskincare.com
Dr. Hauschka: www.drhauschka.com
Dr. Lancer: www.lancerdermatology.com/product_list.php
Dr. Murad: www.murad.com
Egyptian Magic: www.egyptianmagic.com
Epicuren: www.epicuren.com
ESPA: www.espaonline.com
Eucerin: drugstores nationwide
Giorgio Armani Beauty: Sak's Fifth Avenue
Guerlain: www.guerlain.com
IPL Laser: see your dermatologist
Jurlique: www.jurlique.com
Kate Somerville: www.katesomerville.com
Kinara: www.kinara.com
Kinerase: www.kinerase.com
Lancôme: www.lancome.usa.com
Mama Mio: www.mamamio.com
Neutrogena: drugstores nationwide
Nicci: www.aroma1.com
Olay Beauty: drugstores nationwide
Philosophy: www.sephora.com
Physicians Formula: www.physiciansformula.com
Preparation H: drugstores nationwide
Skinceuticals: www.skinceuticals.com
Smashbox: www.smashbox.com
Sonya Dakar: www.sonyadakar.com
Triluma: available by prescription only
Urban Decay: www.sephora.com
Vanicream: www.vanicream.net
Weleda: www.weleda.com and Whole Foods
    Market and Target

Hotels and Spas with Pregnancy Programs, Treatments, and/or Babymoon Packages

LUXURY HOTEL SPAS
The Four Seasons Chicago: www.fourseasons.com
Mandarin Oriental: www.mandarinoriental.com
Peninsula Hotels: www.peninsula.com
Ritz-Carlton: www.ritzcarlton.com
Trump Hotels and Resorts: www.trump.com
Las Ventanas al Paraiso: www.lasventanas.com
W Hotels: www.starwoodhotels.com/whotels/index.html

DESTINATION SPA RESORTS
Babymoon packages: www.babymoonguide.com
Boulders Resort & Golden Door Spa:
    www.theboulders.com
Canyon Ranch: www.canyonranch.com
Casa Madrona Hotel & Spa: www.casamadrona.com
The Greenhouse Spa: www.thegreenhousespa.net
Estancia La Jolla Hotel & Spa:
    www.estancialajolla.com
Miraval Arizona Luxury Resort and Spa:
    www.miravalresort.com
Ojai Valley Inn & Spa: www.ojairesort.com

DAY SPAS
Amomi Pregnancy Wellness ~ Spa:
    www.amomispa.com
Barefoot & Pregnant:
    http://spa.barefootandpregnant.com
Bliss Spa: www.blissworld.com
Contour Day Spa: www.contourspaplantation.com
Edamame Spa: www.edamamespa.com
Elizabeth Arden Red Door Spas:
    www.reddoorspas.com
Exhale Spas: www.exhalespa.com
The Mezzanine Spa: www.mezzaninespa.com
The Mommy Spa: www.themommyspa.com
Spa Space: www.spaspace.com

Miscellaneous
Britax: www.britax.com
Diaper Genie: www.target.com
Dr. Brown bottles: www.target.com
Dreft: drugstores nationwide
Lansinoh: drugstores nationwide
Lilypadz: www.target.com
Pedialyte: drugstores nationwide
Snap-N-Go Stroller: www.target.com

ABOUT THE AUTHOR

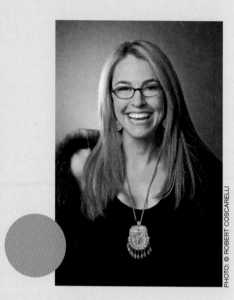

AMY TARA KOCH is a Chicago-based freelance journalist and trend aficionado. She contributes to *Town & Country*, *The New York Times, American Way, INC, Travel + Leisure,* DailyCandy, The Huffington Post, and *Child*. Koch has also served as style columnist for *The Chicago Tribune,* fashion and beauty editor for iVillage, and host for THE INC LIFE, an online trend program for *INC* magazine. Koch is also the trend reporter for NBC (WMAQ-TV) and a style expert for *Vogue* and *USA Today*.

In addition to her media presence, Koch is a speaker and consultant whose clients include Macy's, P&G, Unilever, Frederic Fekkai, Starbucks, Foote Cone & Belding, and the McDonald's Corporation.

Koch has also held posts at *Paper, Mademoiselle,* and BCBG Max Azria and has handled celebrity relations, events, and fashion marketing for luxury brands such as Allure, Van Cleef & Arpels, Bottega Veneta, Bobbi Brown Cosmetics, and Sony.

Koch lives in Chicago with her husband, Peter Gottlieb, and their daughters, Isabella and Brette.

ABOUT THE ILLUSTRATOR

ANNIKA WESTER was born in Sweden but currently resides in Paris. Her work has appeared in fashion publications such as *Glamour Germany, Elle UK, Vogue Nippon, The Wall Street Journal,* and *Seventeen*. She has also worked with Clairol, Kiehl's, MAC Cosmetics, and Anna Sui.